A CHANGING FACES PUBLICATION

Changing Faces:
The Challenge of Facial Disfigurement

James Partridge was born and brought up in Bristol and went to school at Clifton College. In 1970, at the age of eighteen, he was seriously facially burned in a car accident. For several years he underwent extensive plastic surgery at Queen Mary's Hospital, Roehampton, London. During this time he read Politics, Philosophy and Economics at University College, Oxford, and obtained his degree in 1975. Having experienced health care as a patient, he became interested in health care worldwide, and went on to do an M.Sc. in medical demography at the London School of Hygiene and Tropical Medicine. He then worked in health service research and medical education as a health economist – first at St Thomas's Hospital and then at the Unit for the Study of Health Policy at Guy's Hospital.

He married in 1978 and moved to his wife's home island of Guernsey where they lived for 14 years with their three children. They set up a dairy farm with 70 head of Guernsey cattle. He combined farming with teaching A-level economics and was active in local environmental issues, current affairs and broadcasting.

Following the favourable reception given to this book, he launched the charity Changing Faces two years later and is its Chief Executive Officer. He now combines the development of the charity's innovative rehabilitation programmes for those with disfigurements with research, fund-raising and media work. He lives and works in London and Guernsey.

James Partridge

Changing Faces
The Challenge of Facial Disfigurement

A CHANGING FACES PUBLICATION

A CHANGING FACES PUBLICATION

First published by Penguin Group
27 Wrights Lane, London W8 5TZ, England
Published in Penguin Books 1990

Second Edition: Published by Changing Faces, 1994
27 Cowper St, London EC2A 4AP, England

Third Edition: Published by Changing Faces, 1997
1 & 2 Junction Mews, London W2 1PN, England

Fourth Edition: Published by Changing Faces, 2003
1 & 2 Junction Mews, London W2 1PN, England

Fifth Edition: Published by Changing Faces, 2006
The Squire Centre, 33-37 University Street, London WC1E 6JN, England

Typeset by DP Photosetting, Aylesbury, Bucks
Printing by Werner Söderström Osakeyhtio
Cover Design: Christopher Binding, Bristol, England
Cover Photograph: George Cathro

CONTENTS

ACKNOWLEDGEMENTS

Many people have encouraged me to write this book, and I cannot possibly mention them all. I would like to thank all those friends who so freely and honestly replied to my request for their reactions to my disfigurement. Their letters were a wonderful source of material about how disfigured people are perceived in the public eye, and an insight into their personal thoughts and those of their children.

The support of my immediate family has always been crucial and unhesitating, not least in providing a ready stream of ideas and criticism for this book. A special thank you for David and Sue, Alison and Clare.

Mr John Clarke, Senior Plastic Surgeon at Queen Mary's Hospital, Roehampton, was kind enough to lend me some excellent reference books and give me the benefit of his considerable experience in treating facially burned people. Ruth Clarke, Senior Burns Sister at Queen Mary's, who was a junior nurse when I was a patient there, has been invaluable as an adviser and an enthusiast for this project. In my view, these two (unrelated) professionals are an excellent example of how to operate a sensitive and caring burns unit.

I must also mention my gratitude to Paddy Downie for encouraging me to write this book and for her tremendous help on the technical chapters, and to Pam Dix of Penguin for keeping faith with me after totally rejecting the first draft!

Closer to home, I could not possibly have undertaken this work without the conscientious and unquestioning spirit shown by Andrew Chandler, who looked after the farm (often in the mud and rain) while I was writing and thinking (in comparative warmth and comfort indoors). The natural exuberance of our three children, Simon, Charlotte and Harriet, filled the house with noise and laughter, and kept me cheerful while writing the difficult bits. Most of all, my wife, Carrie, has been a tower of strength throughout: editing and typing numerous drafts, cajoling and badgering me when necessary, and always believing that I could finish the book. I am a very lucky man . . .

A PERSONAL NOTE

I was eighteen years old, just about to leave school and planning to go to university after working and travelling for nine months. It was a cold, drizzly night in early December 1970. I was driving a Land Rover to north Wales with a party of school friends for a weekend's walking. The road north from Chepstow joins a dual carriageway just outside the town of Usk. The signs seemed misleading, the left-hand bend came up rather suddenly, and before we knew it the Land Rover had toppled over and was skidding on the driver's side across the carriageway.

Someone swore. I had time to think that we'd have to get a crane to set the vehicle on its wheels again. Then there was a whoosh as the petrol tank exploded, and flames were everywhere. The others clambered out of the back – largely unscathed – but I was lying in the flames, luckily still conscious thanks to my seat belt, and it took me a few seconds to escape. I was on fire.

My life was probably saved by the prompt action of an ex-nurse and her fiancé in the following car; she sacrificed her white fur coat to keep me warm, and their evening out, to drive me at speed in their car to hospital. After ten days in intensive care at St Lawrence's Hospital, Chepstow, I was moved to Queen Mary's Hospital, Roehampton, suffering from severe facial and body burns.

During the next four months I was bed-bound and gradually discovering what a dramatic change had befallen me. At first I still had hope that I would quickly be able to pick up my life where I had temporarily left it. But the permanence of my facial injuries, my seemingly incapacitated left hand and severely weakened legs became all too obvious.

Facial disfigurement is not easily mastered, I discovered. My present facial looks were created over the course of four years, as I went through a long series of plastic surgery operations. During that time I managed to take up my university place, and in the vacations I went to hospital for more surgery. Beyond surgery I determined to live as full and active a life as I would have done had I not been disfigured.

The time spent in hospital had given me an interest in health care, illness prevention and health promotion. After university I decided to specialize in this area, and I took up a job in a London teaching hospital as a 'health economist'. I later moved to Guy's Hospital, London, to work more in the field of health promotion – researching health care and NHS management, and trying to teach medical students and community medicine specialists the rudiments of economics. Any initial embarrassment I – or they – had over someone looking for me being a lecturer was soon dissipated, as the students became interested in the subject of health economics as well as in discovering, often for the first time, what it could be like to be a long-term patient and the recipient of their medical care.

I met my future wife in the middle of 1977. We were married the next year, and soon after we decided to move to her native Island of Guernsey. We have spent several years establishing a dairy farm with a fine herd of pedigree Guernsey cows. In addition, I teach A-level Economics to sixth formers at the local girls' school. We have a family of three children, many good friends, and are both actively involved in many aspects of island life.

The inspiration to write this book came from my belief that the many victims of fires and other disasters, big and small, could benefit from a general guide to rehabilitation after severe facial injury. Twenty years of facial disfigurement have shown me that it is not just the victims but also their friends and families, those who care for them in hospital and all those who come into contact with them in their daily life who would gain from greater understanding. I hope the book will kindle enthusiasm and drive for successful rehabilitation and break down some of the taboos and unease surrounding facial disfigurement.

I have never intentionally used my disfigurement as an excuse for being treated in a special way. Instead I have tried to cultivate the art of wearing my new face with pride. Above all, my face has opened new doors in my understanding of life and people. I refuse to see it as a handicap.

A Note for the Second Edition

Since these pages were written, my life has been hugely affected by the reactions of others to reading them. Two people in particular, one an eminent plastic surgeon mentioned in these pages, the other an academic psychologist who has specialised in the study of facial disfigurement, sowed the seed of an idea. At its heart was the vision to establish a new sort of rehabilitation for those affected by disfigurements, whatever their cause, whether from accident, birth, cancer treatment, a skin condition, a facial paralysis or for any other reason.

The idea started to develop while I was milking cows; the great kindness of one benefactor and the generosity of many others allowed me to take it further, and finally, in 1992, the charity, Changing Faces, came to life. It is principally a 'training ground' to which people, young and not-so-young, can come to 'learn how to cope with disfigurement'. We place particular emphasis on the communication skills required to deal with other people's reactions to the disfigurement. Changing Faces also aims to raise public awareness of the issues that facially disfigured people face every day.

My family has supported me wonderfully throughout this process of change and when it became difficult to keep the farm going, we went through the agony of selling the cows and eventually leaving Guernsey. I thank them for their fortitude.

July 1994

'Goodbye, till we meet again!' Alice said as cheerfully as she could.

'I shouldn't know you again if we did meet,' Humpty Dumpty replied in a discontented tone, giving her one of his fingers to shake: 'you're so exactly like other people.'

'The face is what one goes by, generally,' Alice remarked in a thoughtful tone.

'That's just what I complain of,' said Humpty Dumpty. 'Your face is the same as everybody has – the two eyes, so' (marking their places in the air with his thumb) 'nose in the middle, mouth under. It's always the same. Now if you had the two eyes on the same side of the nose, for instance – or the mouth at the top – that would be some help.'

'It wouldn't look nice,' Alice objected. But Humpty Dumpty only shut his eyes, and said, 'Wait till you've tried.'

From Alice Through the Looking Glass by Lewis Carroll

Changing Faces – A Journey of Reconstruction

If we ever stop to think about it, most of us share a common and simple idea of what constitutes a 'normal' face. Most people have normal faces, which can include the stunningly beautiful as well as the average quite plain and unremarkable face. A few people have dominating blemishes – a hooked nose or a large wart, for example – but even if their features are considered 'ugly', they still fall within the category of having normal faces.

Occasionally we come across someone with a face that is so unusual, so disfigured, that we call it 'abnormal'. It has been severely scarred, deformed or blemished. What could have happened? Does it mean the underlying personality has been similarly damaged and rendered abnormal too? How could he* bear to walk around looking so odd? Couldn't plastic surgery help?

This book is about what happens if and when you (or someone you know) suffer serious facial damage and are consequently disfigured for life. Its message is that it is possible for you, your family and friends to come to terms with your changed and blemished face. Facially disfigured people *can* walk down a street, get a job, have a normal social life.

Becoming facially disfigured for life brings a whole host of challenges and new battles, but, most of all, it is accompanied from the first day with a fear of being 'written off'. You feel that because your face looks so obviously unattractive, and maybe even suspicious, people will judge your personality on this basis and take you literally 'at face value'. Strangely enough, the fear of being taken just at face value actually haunts even the most handsome people. Robert Redford, the successful American film

---

* Here, and throughout the book, 'he' or 'she' could equally apply.

actor, has experienced a similar problem. He was recently quoted as saying, 'I've had a problem with my looks right from the start. It's easy for people to write me off as being no more than my looks.'

The process of coming to terms with facial injury or deformity – what I have called 'changing faces' – is ultimately about showing to the world that your face alone is in no way indicative of your real worth as a human being. Just because you have been unlucky enough to suffer facial damage is no reason to suppose that you are less of a person. Indeed, quite the reverse may be the case, because your experience will probably make you a better and a wiser peson. You certainly have no reason to write yourself off.

In some respects, it is interesting to compare the psychological challenge posed in changing faces with the problem of someone wearing a pair of glasses for the first time. When you begin to wear glasses, you may find you are the subject of considerable interest and comment among your circle of friends and social contacts. You feel rather odd and may try to remove the new glasses as often as possible, for fear that you will seem rather different and conspicuous with them on (despite the fact that this draws even more attention to them, and, in any case, they help you to see better). In public places, you will be sure that people are looking at you because of the glasses; 'How odd that person looks', you imagine them saying. But over a few weeks you will attune yourself completely to the new identity and will get used to being seen as a glasses-wearing person. Maybe you will even use the glasses to give yourself a more learned or sophisticated image.

Putting on glasses changes your outward appearance a fraction, and you may, as a result, slightly change your estimation of yourself. Wearing the mask of facial disfigurement will produce much more dramatic changes, both outwardly and in your own self-image. You have to adjust to these and find new ploys to cope with meeting strangers. Perhaps most daunting of all are public places, but you can find ways of surviving even these. I hope this book will help.

Many facially damaged people wish they could walk around with a placard announcing, 'My face may be a mess but it is no reflection of my personality', or words to that effect. That is the message you have to convey somehow. This book is not going to offer any miracle cures, just as plastic surgery doesn't provide a total answer. 'Changing faces', in the fullest sense, means being able to enjoy living with, and in spite of, your disfigurement. It doesn't happen overnight. You have to work very hard at it.

No one who is injured facially can regain their composure without immense help, support and encouragement from many different people and organizations. Your long process of recovery will rely on the unconditional willingness of your family and friends to 'stay with you', and you will, like me, owe them a tremendous and unrepayable debt of gratitude. Equally, hospital and other professional carers will display so much skill and dedication when helping you that they will always have a special place in your thoughts. I hope that they too will find this book a useful aid to their work.

The Challenge of Changing Faces

Whatever your particular facial impairment, be it a birthmark, unsightly scars, palate deformity, skin grafting, the aftermath of cancer or some other blemish, you face two interrelated problems in regaining your equilibrium. You may have to undergo considerable hospitalization in order to have a presentable physical appearance reconstructed. At the same time, and for the rest of your life, you will have to learn how to live with an odd, conspicuous and damaged face.

In this book I have chosen to deal with these two aspects of changing faces separately: facial reconstruction in Part 1 and psychological and social rehabilitation in Part 2. These two elements are mutually reinforcing: the success of your progress in facial reconstruction will promote your social recovery, and, conversely, your personal achievements outside hospital may make facial surgery less urgent.

So, whatever the cause of your facial disfigurement, a long and challenging recovery lies ahead. Not only do you have physical healing and surgery to go through, but you must also learn to adapt to a new face, walk with it, talk through it, smile in it, wake up with it, go to work with it . . . None of these activities will be easy until you feel at home with your new face. Initially it may appal you, and your image of yourself may be seriously damaged. What is more, other people may be appalled by it too.

Successfully changing faces amounts to completely facing up to your new face and wearing it in public with pride and confidence, and effectively persuading all those whom you meet that behind your mask is a perfectly normal person with normal human emotions and mental abilities.

Changing faces is a process that will change you. You will take on new ways of behaving, new ways of relating to people and new attitudes to others in similar situations to yourself. There is no blueprint for changing faces successfully – everyone will face his circumstances in his own way. But there are certain very clear ideas and guide-lines that I believe are useful in any recovery.

The transition from first realizing what you have done to your 'old' face to the moment when you really feel happy with your 'new' one is likely to be long and drawn out, maybe taking five to ten years, or more. In some ways, the transformation is never complete, because throughout the rest of your life there will be occasions when, even though you and your immediate circle of family, friends and colleagues have become completely used to it, suddenly your face is once again 'on trial', as you meet a new situation. You will never be able to hide from your disfigurement.

Throughout the book I have used the experience of facial disfigurement after fire or heat as the background for discussing the process of changing faces. My own experience of surviving a serious car fire and sustaining severe facial burns illustrates some themes, but this is very definitely not an autobiographical tale. My intention throughout is to inform you about the problems and challenges that lie ahead, to give you ideas and insights into how you might tackle them and, above all, to inspire you to join me on the journey of changing faces.

The Mask of Disfigurement

Facing up to your disfigurement means putting on your new face as if it were just a mask. In burns units all the hospital staff and visitors wear sterile masks to prevent the risk of infection. For many weeks burned patients will see faces covered by these masks: only the eyes show. And it comes as quite a shock to see the rest of a nurse's or doctor's face after months of looking at eyes only! There is a strange irony in this: you lie there building friendships and trust with people whom you recognize only by eyes, and the rest of their face is completely irrelevant. Then you look at yourself in the mirror and realize quite quickly that your own face will always be behind a mask.

You have accepted and related to all these masked people over the weeks and months of hospitilization. You have learned to read their mood and reactions by the look in their eyes or the lines on their forehead. The faces covered up by the masks are irrelevant at the time. They could even have been disfigured. What matters is their laughter, the light in their eyes, their care, advice and encouragement. As a disfigured person, you have to learn to wear the mask of disfigurement like a hospital mask: make sure that your mask does not obscure or dim your real self. If anything, you have to make your real self that much more conspicuous, just as the nurse who wears a mask will accentuate eye movements and style of speech. In other words, you have to come out of your introspection and adopt a new, more outgoing posture.

This advice may seem to run so counter to your natural instincts, which may be to shut yourself away, that you may find it hard to take. Changing faces does involve real change. It isn't just a simple matter of discarding one face and putting on another, everything else unchanged. No, the moral of the hospital mask is that even blank, white sterile masks are full of expression, care and affection, because the wearers deliberately choose to show these things in non-facial ways. You have to learn to do so too, using the whole of your new disfigured face.

The journey of changing faces is long and arduous, pitted with disappointment and disillusion, but do not be disheartened. You will also enjoy many moments of laughter and happiness, and will be profoundly grateful to many people who will help you to wear your mask with confidence and pride. Your journey will begin, as mine did, with the shock of looking at yourself in a mirror. This is the starting-point for changing faces.

PART 1

Reconstructing Your Face

CHAPTER 1

Looking at Your Face in the Mirror

Your face feels puffy, sore, bruised; your facial expressions are restricted – you can't smile: your sight is blurred. You lie still and wonder, what have I done? Could it be serious? I never thought this sort of thing would happen to me. What must I look like?

Facing up to the mirror for the first time is a vital step in changing faces – and getting used to looking in a mirror day by day is one of the biggest hurdles in the process of recovery. Can you ever accept that the reflection you see is really 'you'? It is an alien and unfamiliar sight, and there are few recognizable land-marks: your eyes see out in the same way, but your mouth, nose, chin and cheeks are different and rather unsightly.

The image that you see in the mirror is your new exterior – it is you in the eyes of the rest of humanity. Your identity has changed. Now you will need a new passport photo. But, more importantly, your internal picture of yourself will gradually change in the weeks and months to come.

Accepting and taking on this new image is not at all easy. But the transition can be made less traumatic if your first oppor-tunities to look at yourself are well timed and accompanied by positive messages from all around.

When you severely injure your face or have it operated on (for cancer, for example), you may not want to get out a mirror immediately to inspect the damage. You will probably have an inkling that you have done something quite serious to it, and this will be confirmed by the reactions you observe in your friends or family in the early days and weeks. These visitors to your hospital bed will not be able to hide their shock and concern – you will see it in their eyes (if, that is, they can bear to look at you).

It is ultimately your decision as to when you do look at yourself in a mirror again, and you may postpone the moment for weeks, even months. Some facially injured people never really come to terms with looking in a mirror ever again – they cannot stand the sight of their distorted and devastated features. They yearn for their lost looks and totally reject their new ones.

This chapter looks at how to prepare yourself for the shock of the mirror and predicts that you will experience many dark and gloomy hours afterwards. But this inevitable despair can give way to an honest reassessment of yourself that is the best hope for the future. How other people, especially your close relations, will react when they see you for the first time after your injury is the subject of the next chapter.

Getting Ready to Look in the Mirror

There are very rarely mirrors in a hospital ward for facially injured people. This is quite a sensible precaution, because there is definitely a right time and a wrong time to look at your face after an accident or major cancer operation. As there are no mirrors available, that moment can be chosen by the nursing and other staff with the co-operation of your family. This sounds as if you, the injured party, are to be kept out of the decision, but there is a very good reason for this. If your general mood is depressive and down-hearted, the moment of first looking at your new face is guaranteed to make your state of mind worse and will probably slow down your physical healing. If, on the other hand, the nursing staff in particular use their considerable experience in choosing the right moment, your recovery will not go into reverse. This is not to say that looking into the mirror for the first time can ever be less than a shattering experience, but it has been proved in many instances that the timing of that first glimpse may critically affect your entire recovery.

Obviously, in some facial injuries only a few days will elapse before you are allowed access to a mirror: for example, in car accidents causing cuts and bruises. But the greater the severity of the facial wounds, the longer in general will be the delay. In extreme cases patients have been known to wait up to three months after being burned before discovering their new looks. I doubt whether it actually pays to wait that long, because the time-lag so distances you from facing up to your new looks that the shock might be all the greater. Indeed, I think there is a reasonable case for saying that the earlier the patient looks at himself the better, assuming some resilience is shown in the early stages of recovery. Everyone must be assessed individually, and some actually prefer not to even think about it, let alone look at it.

Facially injured people who do refuse or are not interested in looking at their new features – and I was one of them – may be expressing their despair and demoralization about their general circumstances. They may have drifted into a state of chronic depression: their lives seem in shreds and tatters, and hardly worth going on with. Although looking in the mirror may make that despair even more profound, the desperation will start to be faced squarely only once you have looked at your disfigured face. To back away from your image is only putting off the day when you start to accept your new features and persuade others of your worth.

A great deal can be gained by seeing, talking with and being inspired by others who have been facially injured. I was enormously uplifted by seeing and talking to a fellow patient who had rescued a small child from a burning tent and had, in the process, suffered severe facial burns. Although the sight of him (and the child herself) made my stomach turn over, I was so touched by his obvious recovery and bravery that it helped me believe that I could do it too – though I couldn't actually voice that feeling at the time.

Very few facial injuries are sustained on their own. They are usually accompanied by other body damage, and it is often these other wounds that can give you a hint of the extent and type of facial damage you may have to look at. With facial burns there will probably be other burned areas for you to observe, but this may not be the case if you have facial cancer or complicated fractures.

But getting mere hints will be hardly any value when the moment of truth arrives. You will be nervous and anxious about the moment. The strange thing about burns to the face, especially full-thickness burns, is that they feel very much like severe bruising, and it is quite common to think that your face is merely a bit puffy and bruised. You may have been living with the theory that actually you've only slightly bumped yourself (if fractured) or that you are mildly singed (if burned). These ideas may have been reinforced by nursing staff and others apprehensive about how you will react when you see the real picture, and keen to keep you in the dark until an appropriate moment arrives. You will know when you are ready.

Looking in the Mirror

You will not be alone – or shouldn't be – when the mirror is offered for the first time: someone, whether a family member, friend or hospital professional ought to be there. And since this moment of truth may actually be some time after your admission to hospital, you may well want to choose who is with you – a special friend, your parents, a nurse, or anyone to whom you can particularly relate. In many burns units today there are clinical psychologists trained to be present at these sorts of moments. Hopefully, they will have made contact with you earlier in your treatment and so know something of how you are likely to respond to the sight of yourself.

Steel yourself, then do it. Have one quick look. Take the mirror away. Then look again but don't stare at yourself. Get a general impression. Then put the mirror away.

'Is that really me,' shouts your inner voice. Your face's symmetry is grossly distorted. The colour of the skin, the swelling, perhaps the missing parts, the scars and unhealed wounds, the surgical metalwork, the stitches – there is so much that is wrong. And yet it is still you. You know you are still intact behind this mask. Although you may be slightly repulsed, you can't resist looking a bit more. Perhaps you focus on a particular area of your face. It starts to dawn on you that this is a new beginning.

It is at once a shattering, awful, sad second. You will be horrified. It will take your breath away. It will send a shiver down your spine. You may put a brave face on it – 'Oh, it's not that bad' – but later the tears might start to flow.

Coming to terms with your severe facial injury has similarities to the experience of mourning the death of a loved one. When you fully realize that your facial good looks have been lost for ever (even if this is some time after first looking in the mirror), your reaction may be to break down into uncontrollable tears. The experience of becoming disfigured is total, final and unchangeable – and so is bereavement.

This spontaneous outflow of tears is sometimes thought to be a sign of weakness, especially in men, and as a result many will try to stop it. Bottling up the emotion may look brave or stoical at the time, but it will do little good in the long run. Weeping does not have to accompany your first glimpse of your new face, but it is important that you let yourself go at some point in the next days or weeks. Don't be afraid to.

Your Early Reactions to Your New Face

The significance of your changed face may take some hours or days to sink in. This is often because it takes some time to realize that it won't just be all right again in a matter of time. At first you are hopeful about the medical and surgical possibilities ahead, and you persuade yourself that after a course of surgery you will be 'back to normal'. Long-delayed grief will start to surface when you eventually understand the limitations of surgery, and you find that your facial good looks have been irrevocably lost.

Any disbelief you may have at first will be banished in the following days, after you have taken several long inspections of your new face. Mirrors become quite compulsive, as you scrutinize every bump and imperfection. It does gradually sink in: a regular hourly tour of inspection of your facial frontier will help you to become very familiar with its new contours. But not everyone can be so calculated in their response.

When you are feeling very low, as you may well be after first glimpses of yourself, you may think that you shouldn't express your bitterness, disappointment and sorrow. But it is hard to keep a traditional 'stiff upper lip', and eventually your external composure will break, your 'brave face' crack and you hit rock bottom. It's a lousy moment. You are powerless to stop it. But there is often a pay-off some days later, when you realize that the spite and venom had to be expressed, and that it is a relief to have done so.

Emotional reactions to a new face vary immensely among

people. There is no 'perfect response' to be displayed. Everyone has to work out his own way of coming to terms with the shock and the new facts of his life. In these early days, emotions are so confused and mixed up that many patients seem to drift between moods of comparative optimism and ones of complete defeatism and depression. Inside you will probably experience a mixture of the following gut feelings:

Anger. You are furious with yourself for your bad luck, or bad judgement, and with others for not understanding or not caring. You may become quite irrational and abusive to those in the ward, hospital staff and visitors. You feel angry not to have been told earlier what a mess your face is in. You feel cheated and deceived.

Misery. You are tormented by your wretched looks and can't stop the sobbing and the ghastly welling-up of tears in the throat. You don't want to think or talk about the future at all and wallow in the sorrow of the moment. You pile up your agony: the hospital imprisonment, your ruined life, your abysmal prospects, your isolation and friendlessness, your stupidity and bad luck at getting facially injured. You debase yourself and become completely negative in your thinking.

Defeatism. You sink into a mire of silent resignation. You reject all conversation and social contact with anyone who is trying to help you. You switch off all feelings of hope (which perhaps had been buoying you up prior to looking in the mirror) and drift towards sullen resignation: 'What's the point?'

Repulsion. You feel completely divorced from your face. You are physically sick at the sight of your wounds, the blood or the severe bruising. You don't want to look again, and, worse, you don't want anyone else to look at it, because it's so revolting.

Distancing. You try to rationalize your facial problem, to think your way out of it. You become obsessed with finding out everything you can about the wounds and the technical aspects of surgery. You distance your face from your inner self and treat your face as just an object for treatment.

Deception. You continue to persuade yourself that you are only slightly injured and something magical will re-create your facial attractiveness. Others may encourage you in this belief for fear that if they don't, you will lose all your will to recover.

Determination. You feel annoyed at your present predicament and determined not to let the damage to your face interrupt your life. But you know that you may be asking too much of yourself – and others. It is difficult to maintain optimism.

Stoicism. You make every effort to hide your emotional response and pretend to the world that you can easily withstand the pain and bear the inevitable trials of your new predicament. Inside, though, your inner voice is constantly doubting your fortitude, and you know you won't be able to keep up the pretence for long.

Talking about Your Reactions

Your initial reactions to seeing your face may be dispiriting. They may last for hours, days or weeks, depending on a number of other outside factors, chief among them being how much social contact you can rely on. The most important requirement for cultivating a positive attitude out of the desperation you will feel is to have good outlets for talking to others. There is nothing more crucial at this stage than having unconditional conversations with friends and indeed strangers – unconditional in the sense that they accept you as you are, without frills or obligations. Above all, your inevitable feeling that 'with a face like this' you are bound to be socially outcast needs to be refuted by them.

Nowadays staff in wards for the treatment of the facially injured have become more aware of the need for open and frank conversations with patients, but often this is attempted by inappropriate people. Surgeons, for example, can be geniuses at getting some of their patients to speak openly about their feelings. However, not everyone feels at home outpouring his sorrows and anxieties to a high-powered doctor. Ward cleaners or untrained ancillary staff are often much more approachable. I can recall a lovely motherly ward cleaner called Josie who addressed all the patients as 'Darling', stood around and chatted to everyone and was always being chided by her supervisors for her slowness: she was a great listener, and she allowed patients to speak without fear of being misunderstood or judged.

Few people who look at their new facial features are going to start up an intellectual or deep conversation about the significance of their new looks a few moments later. It is not possible to force any spoken reaction. You must find your voice by confiding in someone. Some people find it easier to talk to someone previously unknown – a member of the ward staff, the hospital chaplain, another patient, an unexpected visitor – and they may well reject opening up to their close family. The presence of a social worker or psychologist may prompt you to start the painful process of rediscovering yourself, but these people also get the cold shoulder on occasion.

The irritation that you may feel if someone tries to get you to talk is understandable. Do not be surprised. Pick your own moment, not theirs. Try to appreciate that it is as difficult to counsel the facially injured as it is people who have been severely injured, paralysed or struck down by a disease. It is hard for them to break through your natural resistance and gain your trust. The vital thing for them is not to try to ask you the big questions until a relationship has been created; otherwise the counsellor or friend is liable to meet withdrawal and/or bitterness and will have, in turn, to withdraw.

Hospital staff in daily contact with the facially wounded provide a critical bridge for them. These caring people are not only making your hospitalization as tolerable as possible, they are also treating you from the word go as a whole person. They have their own lives outside the hospital, but they get to know you. And you will get to rely on them – sometimes very heavily indeed.

Whatever your emotional reaction to your new looks, the first step on your road to changing faces is to acknowledge your position, and that comes by communicating your gloom to someone else and sharing your worst fears. The care and empathy of hospital staff, your family and friends will be enormously important: being a good listener is never easy, rarely an ability that can be learned and, in this busy, time-conscious world, an unpractised skill. Finding a good listener allows you to offload your early reactions and thereby start on the road to accepting your new face.

CHAPTER 2

Being Looked at by Your Family

You have looked at your new face. Now you start to watch how your close family and friends who come to visit you in hospital are looking at it, and how they are reacting to it and you. You appreciate that they might find the sight of you difficult to accept, let alone to talk about. How can you make it easier for them?

The first steps in changing faces are taken in the relative security of a hospital ward. Here your social contacts are principally with the people who pay you visits, staying for anything from half an hour to (exhausting) marathon four-hour sittings. They are the first people to show their reactions to your face. They have usually come to help *you*, but you may well find that you have to help them.

You have to work a lot harder at relationships if you are disfigured. As soon as you discover your new facial identity, you have to start finding suitable ways of expressing yourself that do not rely on the face alone. Your family represents the first group of people on whom you will be able to try this out. By watching them, you can learn why they behave as they do towards you, and this will enable you to develop appropriate ways of conveying yourself to others. This process of learning how to interact actually takes many years, but it usually starts in your relationships with your closest family and friends.

The First Reactions of Family and Friends

In many facial accidents or disorders, your spouse, parents, siblings and friends get to see your new looks long before you do yourself. After your first look, you may want to ask questions and discuss an area that they may feel is extremely tender. They may be at a loss to know how to respond to you – 'What can I say that will be of any value?' They are worried that you will be worried if you see them showing their worry ... This is uncharted territory for all concerned.

Relatives and friends of the facially injured find it hard to come to terms with the first sight of facial wounds, and even harder to accept that the wounds are bound to leave disfiguring scars. The assumptions made in the early days after a fire, for example, that all will be back to normal in a few weeks will gradually give way to the discovery that facial disfigurement is for life. Relatives, especially husbands, wives or loved ones, have to make some major adjustments to this truth and, not surprisingly, are sometimes unable to do so.

Just as you find yourself tackling a range of complicated intertwined emotions when confronted with the stark realization that the facial injuries are permanent, so too do relatives and friends experience profound reactions that they may exhibit in a number of ways.

Total commitment. Close family members realize that you will need huge support, and they commit themselves to completely ignoring your facial blemishes and throwing themselves into aiding and assisting you in every possible way. This sort of selflessness is occasionally a front for self-deception or not wanting to face up to the truth, but often it has as its foundation a strong religious faith, a deep empathy with you as a result of some major experience earlier on in life, or a profound bond of love. It is amazing to feel the warmth and totalness of this reaction.

However, total commitment can have drawbacks – it can verge on suffocation. Their 100 per cent willingness to help and aid may inhibit you from actually starting the slow process of acknowledging your grief before facing up to the world again. It can feel as if you are being protected and closeted off from the reality of your predicament. However close and cushioning the much needed support that relatives bring, it must not shelter you from what has happened. A balance has to be struck, and you may feel it necessary to push the close protection away at times.

Sorrow and sympathy. Family and friends feel so wretched and helpless that they offer huge dollops of 'I'm so sorry for you' and

'It must feel awful' and 'I don't know how you can bear it – you're so brave'. The sight of your badly injured face makes them feel so sad that it could have happened to you, and almost guilty that it didn't happen to them. They sit beside you, not daring to tell you any happy pieces of news from the outside world, and almost wanting you to confirm that it feels as bad as it looks – because knowing this will confirm their sadness.

This is a very understandable reaction to the sight of ghastly facial wounds, because they do probably look far worse than they feel (especially when you take into account how sophisticated pain control is nowadays). The trouble is that this show of sympathy may allow and even encourage an inward-looking and self-pitying attitude on your part that can have an insidious and undermining effort on your recovery. As you start to feel sorry for yourself, you question your ability to 'be brave' for very much longer ... Although you may be grateful for the messages of sympathy, you may find them hard to take because they exacerbate your problem. You may have to say directly to the oversympathetic that you are OK and confident of recovery – even if you have your doubts.

Avoidance. The feeling of inadequacy about what to say or how to act towards the facially damaged person drives some to varying degrees of avoidance strategies – from totally staying away to compromise visiting (where the visitor makes no real effort to communicate but merely inquires about your welfare, hardly listens to your reply and then departs). This 'inadequacy' response is unfortunately compounded by the common feeling of guilt about not doing more or saying more, and the consequence is even less confidence about visiting.

It is important that the facially injured person takes action to make the awkward visitor feel more at ease. Avoidance is made more likely if there is no comeback from the injured party. You must try to find ways of reassuring visitors, especially those who are finding it hard to know where to look. Full recovery from facial injury (in other words, successfully changing faces) will often call for you to make a major effort to communicate your personality and help other people to face your face.

Part of the reason for avoidance is the visitor's feeling that he has no answers to your predicament – and that there aren't any obvious answers available. If you want to bridge the 'avoidance' gap, I think you have to show first that you can read the visitor's mind and understand how he may be feeling about you, and secondly try to persuade him that you believe there are ways of coping – 'After all, look at X who manages in a wheelchair.'

Soul-searching. Many relatives go through a heart-aching analysis of their reaction to your injury. They agonize (though not usually in your presence) about how to communicate with you, and unfortunately this may lead them to become acutely self-conscious when they visit you. They are aware of their natural instinct to stand back from contact but at the same time desperately want to be of some value.

The agonizing self-consciousness these visitors show is often very obvious to you even from behind their surgical masks. You may well share their uncertainty as to how to adjust to your face, and you may therefore appreciate their difficulty. This coincidence of uncertainty between you and them can be the opportunity to open up a discussion about how you can carry your face around in public and about how they think people will react to it. I have found that people are usually so relieved to be talking about it that they can often offer really useful ideas for your recovery.

The most encouraging thing about such frank conversations is that you discover that you can still have good friends – indeed, that your old friends are still with you. And **they** discover that you haven't changed that much, and if so, for the better. In this way, you have helped them out of their dilemma about how to treat you, and they have given you ideas and encouragement – a two-way process with communication drawing you together.

Rejection. Some visitors will experience such strong revulsion at the sight of your facial wounds, especially facial burns, that they will be incapable of relating to you at all. They find that they are ashamed to be associated with you, and they avoid your company at all costs. This is a very painful situation: occasionally it occurs between marriage partners, with devastating consequences for everyone (including hospital staff). Sometimes the rejection lasts for a long time and is untreatable, but in many instances, close family can be brought into a helping role.

Rejection is not simply about the horror of your facial looks. There are usually more fundamental causes that have come to the surface as a result of your facial injury. Your misfortune is the trigger for you to be outcast by your family. If, for example, they perceive that your facial problem is in some sense self-inflicted or if your hospitalization has created a huge domestic crisis, latent family conflicts may surface. In these circumstances, professional counselling and assistance is imperative. An objective third party must try to arbitrate and act as a go-between. The healing of these family rifts will be a prerequisite to successful facial rehabilitation.

In many instances, relatives and friends will waver between different shades of these various responses. Just because they appear to be soul-searching one day does not mean they will be in a similar frame of mind the next time they visit. So you will have to constantly adjust your responses to them too.

Nobody could suggest that discovering that a loved one's face is permanently disfigured is anything other than a ghastly experience, and it is therefore crucial that the whole range of hospital staff should be very sensitive to the needs, questions and anxieties of family and close friends. Changing faces depends so much on family encouragement and staying-power that every effort must be made to help them to adopt a forward-looking approach.

Mourning the loss of the good looks of a lover, son, daughter, brother, sister, parent or friend must give way to a robust refusal to look back to the handsome or pretty face of old. That perfection has been dulled, but ahead is a major challenge: facing the world with an abnormal face. For relatives the challenge is to be willing and ready to be seen with you in public, to believe that you can recover your poise, if not your looks, and to reaffirm that despite all your horrible injuries you are still the same lover, son, daughter . . . They can't take up that challenge without your help.

Getting Help from the Professionals

Hospital staff, especially social workers and counsellors, have the responsibility for trying to put the close family of the facially injured back on the rails. Despite the enormity of this task, the job of your surgeon is even more fundamental. The surgeon should have qualifications in 'communication skills' along with his medical training, and set the tone for your facial rehabilitation by being available for lengthy conversations when necessary and by providing realistic judgements about your outlook. You and your family have to feel some rapport with your surgeon – and he with you. The ability of the surgeon to 'click' with parents, spouses, etc., often makes the difference between a slow, uninspired recovery and a hopeful but realistic one. There is a delicate balance to be struck between being excessively optimistic (and then failing to live up to expectations) and offering unduly depressing forecasts (even if they may be closer to the truth). The surgeon must make a decision, often within a few minutes of meeting your immediate family, as to how to pitch his advice and prognosis.

Having chosen a line of argument, it is incredibly important that the surgeon then liaises well with the nursing staff, because they more than anyone will field the daily and regular questions about progress and specific facial damage. Relatives must be able to talk freely with nursing staff and discover as much relevant information as possible – within the guide-lines laid down by the surgeon. Sometimes lines of communication get crossed and much pain and confusion results. Relatives get one line of thinking from one professional and a contradictory one from another, resulting in loss of confidence for all concerned.

Burns units today give considerable attention to the psychological care of the facially injured patient's family. Much of this falls on the social worker assigned to the case. Many of the fears expressed by the family are ones that the patient will experience concerning his acceptability in public places and the chances of the face ever being restored to something vaguely acceptable.

There are no straight or perfect answers to these problems. The families of the facially wounded have to appreciate this and hopefully give undivided support to the healing and restorative effort, fraught with ups and downs as it will inevitably be. The 'new looks' may be unappealing, but there are ways and means of living with them.

Ploys for Visiting the Facially Injured

'What can I say? What should I say?' These are common anxieties when visiting a facially injured friend in hospital. Although there is no perfect formula for hospital visiting, it is useful to go into a hospital armed with some ideas for comforting or consoling.

The first thing is to be prepared for a shock. Facial injuries are often very unpleasant to look at, but remember that behind the wounds is a confused but generally alert mind, possibly somewhat sedated to prevent excessive pain. There are no magic words that you can utter. Say something honest and don't be afraid to ask direct questions, where appropriate. Do look at the face and eyes in front of you, however painful that may be to you. But try not to stare blankly!

The chances are that your disfigured friend will want to talk, but possibly not about a subject you would expect. Patients may need to be distracted by good and bad news, gossip and chat from the outside world. They want to keep in touch with what is going on. So talk about your plans – even for holidaying in the sun! Bring sunshine and humour into the ward. Don't worry that this sounds rather frivolous. The distracting effect of talking normally with friends greatly boosts the patient's morale at the time, even if afterwards there is a tendency to feel rather deflated.

Don't try to force the conversation into difficult areas where the patient may think he has to give away secrets about his feelings. Periods of silence are important: they give the patient a chance to start a new conversation or ask a leading question. They also allow the patient time to adjust to being with other people with his new looks.

Try to listen, encourage, empathize – but do not patronize. In other words, try to avoid saying things that sound empty and encouraging like 'Oh you are brave' or 'I couldn't bear what you're going through'. These will set the patient's teeth on edge, because he has no choice but to undergo the treatment, the dressings and the operations. Bravery is shown where there is a choice.

The major message for visitors is to convey that they are interested. To know that someone cares that you are incarcerated in a hospital ward, miles from family and home, is immensely gratifying in itself. It is even more comforting for the facially disfigured, because they may well be suffering from the 'I'm written off' syndrome, whereby no one could possibly be interested in them, their thoughts and hopes.

Changing faces involves more than just looking at yourself and accepting that 'That's me'. You will need to talk over and over the events in which you suffered injury. This is a very necessary part of recovery from any accident of whatever kind, whether facial or not. You have got to get a lot of the tension of the event out of your system, and this will place heavy demands on any listeners, especially if they are struggling to appreciate what has happened. You have to learn how to look into other people's eyes and see their reactions to you and then respond accordingly. Your close family and friends visiting you in hospital will offer you the first opportunity to start practising these lessons.

CHAPTER 3

Facing up to the Cause of Your Injuries

Being facially injured is a devastating experience. Whatever the cause of it, that moment of fire, explosion or other shock is the start of a life that will be very different from the one you had imagined or hoped for. It may be many months, or even years, before you can dispassionately recall the details of the event and talk about them without feeling the emotion of the moment running away with you. For many, the early days and weeks after a fire or major disaster are punctuated by nightmares and horrible memories.

You may well want to forget the moments of your accident for ever, but that is impossible. Somehow you have to face up to what happened: successfully changing faces demands that you do not look back with bitterness but manage to reconcile yourself to your new circumstances. Such a reconciliation will be made easier if you frankly and openly go over the details of your disaster. There may be aspects of it that raise questions about your own or someone else's competence, and the resulting anger may linger and cloud your recovery. Even if you were completely to blame, and this is unlikely since there are nearly always contributory factors, you can still take on your new face as a new chapter in your life, once you have admitted your failing to yourself. But if you hate yourself, or somebody else, your facial injury will be an intolerable load that you will neither shake off nor learn to carry with dignity.

In this chapter I have concentrated on the experience of being in a fire, and I have attempted to bring a reflective slant to what is a really horrific memory. Anybody who is burned has to come to terms with flames and fires, be able to enjoy a bonfire party on a moonlit night and stand warm beside the inferno enjoying the heat . . . Recalling the experience of fire can help you to put it into perspective. Whatever the cause of your disfigurement, you have to be honest with yourself.

Being on fire is unforgettable. You will recall those seconds with crystal clarity for the rest of your life. In fact, those who don't remember usually don't survive: fire strikes so fast that if you are knocked unconscious, you stand very little chance. The human body can tolerate only a few seconds in the intense heat and airlessness of a hot fire.

Unforgettable those seconds may be, but they are not ones you will replay with any pleasure. Physically, fires do maim the body in very unpleasant ways, though surprisingly many people caught in flames feel little or no pain. But fires also have other character-istics that, when added together, make fire one of the most feared and terrifying of all natural forces.

Fires are so sudden: the dividing line between a controlled fire and one that is out of control is paper thin. Whether the fire is in a kitchen, a car, at a bonfire party or a football match, the flash of flames and the searing heat come out of the blue. And fire is totally undiscriminating – it burns anything in its path and reduces it to ashes.

There is no getting away from the nightmare of being in a fire, or of being a witness to one. Your appreciation of life itself will have changed. However awful you think you look now, just being alive after a fire is worth rejoicing at. You will know how slender is the thread that keeps us alive and how it feels to be close to personal extinction. It is worth remembering how precious life is when you question whether you can ever enjoy anything in the same way as you did 'before'. The fire is a watershed, a change in the direction and meaning of your life.

Being on Fire

Speed of reaction to a fire or scald is absolutely vital to survival. And yet the experience of many who have been caught in a fire is that the element of surprise actually disables you. So stunned are you to find yourself in the flames that you are literally immobilized. There is a momentary inability to do anything – and in those few seconds the damage can be done. In my own case, when suddenly faced by flames, I felt a numbness to action. This was followed by an inexplicable but life-saving surge of energy to get out of the suffocating fire, which gave way to a feeling of delirious elation at being alive. Thus within a single minute I experienced a quite staggering range of emotions.

People ask me, 'What was it like?' Words can hardly describe being on fire: painless, breath-taking, all-embracing, hot, life-threatening, 'Help!' Thinking is not really coherent in the instant of inferno. You know instinctively that your life is in the balance. For a split second you think of loved ones. There are voices and screams. The heat is totally enveloping and stifling. Air is desperately short – rather like being breathless under water.

To escape the flames is to feel total release from hell. Fresh air is gasped in. Many fires today are compounded by clouds of noxious fumes, and clean air is all the more gratifying. But the feeling of release can prompt extremely dangerous behaviour. I ran round like an idiot with my clothes on fire. I should have rolled on the ground to douse the flames, but I didn't realize I was on fire. Instead I actually fanned the flames leaping from my polo-neck sweater and my jeans. I felt no pain. Indeed, I told my anxious friends that I was just singed.

You are certainly oblivious to the damage you have suffered. My accident happened at night, so the darkness concealed my injuries, but I did not try to look at my hands or burned areas. I was aware of people at the scene looking at me in a worried fashion, but all I felt was a swelling of my face and a numbness in my hands and legs. No agony, very little pain, but gradually I was losing consciousness.

The extent of pain is dependent upon how severe your burns are: the deeper they are, the less painful they will be, because the heat will destroy the nerve-ends in your skin. But your mental pain and acute anxiety may reach very high and uncontrollable levels. People will try to sooth and reassure you, but the terror of the event will keep recurring in your mind – replay after replay will bring back the horror of the moment.

What is so inspirational in so many fires is how onlookers, fire brigade officers and even those already burned are brave enough to try to rescue other badly burned or trapped people from the blaze. Fire is so untouchable that these efforts are acts of heroism

and too often go unrewarded. However, the gratitude that rescued people feel towards their rescuers is unbounded. I, for one,
know that I owe my life to the swift and selfless actions of a
couple, both of whom were total strangers to me.

The Nightmare and the Shock

Survival from fires does not simply bring severe physical injuries.
Psychological trauma is now widely recognized as being almost as
life-threatening. The skills of accident and emergency units in
modern hospitals have advanced so that the physical risks have
been considerably reduced. But there is now a growing interest
in the psychological treatment for the victims (and witnesses) of
major and minor catastrophes – not just infernos but other
incidents too.

Most people who survive will have seen and been deeply
distressed by some awful sights. These will form the stuff of
nightmares and waking flashbacks. Your own wounds may be
involved, but more likely you will be particularly upset by the
suffering of other people, the terror you saw, and the agony that
you were powerless to relieve or prevent. These recurrent images
are characteristic (and perhaps newsworthy) of some of the
survivors of the massive disasters of recent years: the Zeebrugge
ferry sinking or the King's Cross Underground fire. But the
smallest fire or personal tragedy will trigger visions just as
disturbing: the kitchen blaze, an accident involving a small child,
the head-on car smash.

The shock of how quickly and terrifyingly the fire or accident
took place will take some days to work through. For some people,
the shock can be delayed or prolonged. There is now a recognized
psychological condition, Post-Trauma Stress Disorder (PTSD),
which may be the way you react to highly disturbing events.
Psychologists have discovered that people do not just experience
occasional flashbacks and nightmares; they may also show signs
of being affected for many months and even years afterwards.

Typically in PTSD, the long-term reactions are symptoms of
fear that the whole ghastly incident might repeat itself, of hostility
towards other people and of chronic anxiety that you will never
be able to live without the memories. If you do suffer from these

sorts of feelings, it would be best to seek specialist advice from a psychologist. Work with the survivors of Zeebrugge, for example, has indicated that long-term counselling can gradually ease the pain and anxiety.

'If only' . . . and 'Why me?'

Almost immediately after a major personal calamity you will find yourself seeking out someone or something to blame for the disaster. After years of assuming 'It'll never happen to me', you suddenly find that it has happened, and you will want to know why.

Many people look back on their failure to respond quickly enough and bemoan their inadequacy. 'If only I'd moved quicker' is a common expression among the burned. Other victims describe their instant reaction to fire as one of pure panic – and they may also look back in anger and frustration. These feelings of self-blame are often the reason why burned people find telling the story of their fire so very difficult. Reliving the experience seems to highlight their shortcomings in the crisis. There are parts of my own story that I still find it hard to accept and live with: why was I driving at 40 mph rather than 30? Why didn't I react quicker to the misleading temporary signposts before the critical corner? Was I really concentrating?

'If only I hadn't . . .' is also a surprisingly common refrain in burns units. Sometimes it simply refers to having been in the wrong place at the wrong time, in which case there is little real self-blame. The accident is put down as just a chance in a million, an act of God – or divine retribution perhaps. There can be only the eternal question 'Why me?', to which there is really no answer.

But where there is doubt about causes and those responsible, you may attach unwarranted blame to yourself: 'I should have checked that gas fire' or 'Why didn't I get the car serviced?' This self-questioning attitude is part of facing up to the unexpurgated version of events, but taken too far and allowed to become a stick to beat yourself with, it can degenerate into self-rejection and profound depression.

No recovery from fire will be successful if there is a constant looking back to what might have happened if only . . . One of the most important roles for family, friends and hospital staff from the outset is to encourage a forward-looking approach. However bleak that future might look – and this book is determined to diminish that bleakness – looking back and bitterly chiding oneself achieves very little. Bygones are bygones. Someone badly burned who is still bitterly blaming himself many months after the event is trapped in a retarded recovery.

Talking about It

In the immediate aftermath of a major fire, you are unlikely to be sufficiently conscious to take much part in the proceedings: the first forty-eight hours are critical, and your life may be in the balance. You may not be aware of this at all at the time. Indeed, when you do regain consciousness you may well talk about your accident as rather a minor incident, not yet being aware of its significance.

Talking about what happened is such a very cathartic activity that I cannot understate its value. 'Catharsis' is the best word I know to describe it: literally, it is a medical word meaning purgation or cleansing. Talking to people, be they family, hospital staff or complete strangers, enables you to let out all the emotion and feelings you have about the fire – it cleanses you of the drama.

Looking back on it later, you may be surprised at how very openly you spoke in the days after your fire. There are no holds barred – everyone involved loses his reticence. Reluctance to talk is unusual.

But the outpouring of emotion is not a simple, matter-of-fact affair. Far from it. Tears and crying: everyone is very upset by what has happened. Shock affects different people in different ways, but no one should bottle up his shock. Those who do will find that they suffer a delayed reaction.

Unfortunately, there is sometimes a typically British reaction to fire damage: a stiff upper lip is adopted by people who come to see you, and as a result neither you nor they may open your hearts as you want. I think this brings a whole host of difficulties, because the time for you to face up to what actually happened to you and how you felt about it is postponed. Some burns victims require psychotherapy many years later in order to vent their anger or sorrow.

I am not suggesting that you or your family or friends must force a discussion of what happened. But you must not be afraid to express yourself for fear of looking silly or weak. You will lie for many hours, thinking your thoughts, staring at the ceiling. When visitors do come, you will have an opportunity to share your experience with them. This sharing is a very strong bond between people in these early days. You entrust them with some very special personal thoughts, and they in their turn show their concern and hope for you. It's a two-way healing process. Recovering from facial injuries is, in the end, about how well you can communicate with the rest of humanity, in spite of your tarnished face. You can start your journey very early on by choosing to find people to talk to about what happened. They will discover that for all your facial wounds you are still remarkably sane, emotional and, above all, alive.

CHAPTER 4

Being a Patient

Whatever the cause of your facial injury or impairment, your first inkling that something serious has befallen you will be gained from the unlikely and unusual perspective of a hospital bed. Many facial injuries result from split-second tragedies that throw their victims completely out of their habitual lifestyle and into an alien, unknown world of hospitals, medicine and highly technological life-saving skills and equipment.

The abrupt change in your circumstances will not affect only you, however. Your family and close friends may have to make some major sacrifices – even financial ones – to be able to come to visit you, and like you, they may feel shocked and uncertain in the hospital environment.

The physical reconstruction phase of changing faces is almost entirely hospital based. You are destined to undergo sufficient surgery to restore your face to a presentable state. In the process you have to enter into a very special relationship with a hospital and its staff. Your first moments of hospitalization will be important – not just because you will be discovering that you have severely injured yourself, but also because you are entering into a totally new and possibly unnerving psychological situation.

Medical and hospital staff take control of your life. They will be making decisions about your treatment, and you will have very little input into these. Your technical knowledge about surgery, for example, is likely to be too sketchy to be of any value. As a facially injured person on the 'critical' list, you have to rely completely on the experience and skill of medical and nursing staff. Changing faces necessitates releasing control of your destiny to other people – you have to trust them totally.

It is a great help if the medical staff gain the trust of your family and explain your predicament, not least because your next of kin may have to sign consent forms to allow you to be operated upon. How well you and they are informed and taken into the confidence of the medical staff is likely to set the tone for your whole course of treatment. It is tragic to meet patients and their families who have not built a firm relationship with the hospital and staff on whom they depend – usually because of an early lack of communication, both parties being at fault.

If trust can be fostered from an early stage – and this may mean that you become very dependent on the support of a particular member of the hospital staff – your own morale and will-power will be constantly boosted, and your recovery accelerated too. More to the point, however brilliant a surgeon is, or however compassionate are the nursing staff, if they do not gain your respect and trust, things will quickly turn sour. It takes a two-way effort: trust has to be developed.

Regaining Full Consciousness

Once taken into an accident and emergency (casualty) department at a hospital, a burned person will probably have his wounds inspected and dressed in the admission room. Pain killers (analgesia) will be administered in order to minimize the pain that is inevitable and would be intolerable and possibly life-threatening if not controlled. It may be some time before you regain full consciousness.

In facial burns, the swelling around the eyes will often be so great that at first you cannot see anything, and this can last for several days. So your first impressions are of considerable unseen activity around your bed. You will feel stiff and sore, but if the analgesia is effective, numb too. You may find yourself restricted in movements by bandaging. One or two familiar voices may be audible, but, for the most part, the voices and the words are strange and incomprehensible.

Any movement from you will be closely monitored at this stage, and, as soon as you try to move or speak, you will feel a presence beside your bed – a kindly voice, a soothing message: 'Don't worry. X is here to see you when you feel up to it. Try not to move too much. Yes, you will feel rather sore for a while. Is there any pain? I'll get you something for it. Would you like a drink?' These are, in retrospect, very special discovery moments. You are realizing in the course of split seconds that something quite serious must have happened. You probably remember the fire – but what about the others involved? Am I really only singed? Why are my relatives here? Where is 'here'? The questions start to pile up, and yet you are so incapacitated and weakened that you drift in and out of sleep.

It's a strange feeling knowing that someone has walked into your room even though you can't see them. But you don't need to be able to see to sense their concern. Hospital wards are always warm, almost stifling, and you can feel empathy and warmth from visitors too. There is no right way for them to react in these circumstances – just being there brings a wave of goodwill and care. Messages from relatives and friends in these first hours are incredibly significant in shaping one's attitude to the future. Yet all this extraordinary attention is at once both pleasing and alarming. Why *is* there so much concern, you wonder.

This question doesn't really get a straight answer, because in most burns cases it is impossible to really predict your long-term outcome for several days, possibly even weeks. Certainly you will not be informed that the first forty-eight hours are critical to your life, although you will be given an outline of what has happened and helped to concentrate on straightforward, everyday concerns like drinking as much as possible, 'using a bottle' or 'having a bowel movement'.

Drinking with very swollen lips is well nigh impossible. But what are those other terms? They refer to matters that are not much discussed in ordinary conversation, but there is no chance of avoiding them now. Your privacy completely breaks down: bedpans, bed-baths and being spoon-fed become second nature after only a few hours. The hospital vocabulary and way of life are already being adopted.

Nurses are soon recognizable by their voices and their touch. Every hour, it seems, they hunt for a place to take your pulse. You can hear them rattling dishes and bottles, putting up another drip. Blood transfusion into a vein, yes – but for how long? You are totally unable to influence what is being done, you are powerless, a passive receiver – a patient.

It is unpleasant, and yet the extraordinary sensation of being alive is there. You are conscious of the relief. Being alive despite the discomfort feels almost good.

Early recovery from extensive burns does depend strongly on will, *your* will to fight for your life; the larger the body area burned, the more vital it is that you fight. Burns unit staff can provide graphic accounts of this truth: people with horrendously high percentage burns survive, while others with less damage don't – and the difference is often the will. To demoralize a patient by too much pessimism can be dangerous – and this justifies any artificial optimism about your future.

With hindsight, I know that I was given to believe several half-truths: that I would probably be out of hospital in three weeks and able to take up life more or less where I had left off. This fitted well with my belief that I was just bruised or singed, and I swallowed it. My brother recalls his quite unwarranted assumption that, give or take a few weeks, the swellings and puffed-up face would all be under control. Whether or not we were deliberately misled by the hospital staff, it helped me and my family through the early days.

Judging the right mixture of honesty versus fiction in talking to someone badly burned is a specialized skill. Usually the surgeon in charge of you will make some kind of preliminary assessment about your prospects. In fact, he is often unable to accurately predict a future, because it will depend greatly on the depth of the burns and that can be difficult to assess at the beginning. So optimistic prognoses can be justified . . .

Already the language, the clean smell and the routine of the hospital start to impinge on your consciousness. As a result of a sudden accident, from being completely unaware of what goes on behind the swing doors of a hospital, you are now the recipient of highly technical and intensive hospital treatment. Within forty-eight hours swelling around the eyes usually starts to go down, and now you can begin to see the full picture of that treatment: bleeping monitors, nurses in masks, oxygen cylinders and lots of transparent tubes attached to bottles at one end and to your arm at the other. These are known as 'drips' (infusion), as you soon learn, because slowly, at a calculated rate, they infuse fluids, including, if necessary, blood, into your depleted system.

Being able to see again – if your sight has not been permanently damaged – will offer the first chance to view your injuries. Despite regular pain killers being administered, it is usually possible to get some idea of their extent by looking at your body, if it is not heavily bandaged, and by asking questions of the medical staff. But you won't be offered a mirror.

Not being able to see your face at this early stage is a positive advantage. Although it may make the sight of your facial wounds that much more shocking later on, the first minutes and hours of consciousness should not be clouded by the sight of them. This is why there are never mirrors in burns wards.

It is enough to see the reactions of friends and family, even behind their surgical masks; these are very revealing. Their sense of shock at the sight of you lying prostrate, swollen, raw or bandaged is obvious. Many visitors will find it hard to look at all; they literally don't know where, or how, to look; they will fuss with the flowers or look out of the window or talk to others in the room.

Being a Patient Patient

Burns and plastic surgery treatments for facial injuries, in common with treatments for other sorts of facial damage, are never completed quickly. The shattering first few days of hospitalization soon become weeks and months, and your full course of plastic surgery will probably go on intermittently for several years. In the process you will find yourself increasingly ruled by the institutional features of the hospital – the routines and the rules – and the formality of carer-cared-for relationships. Your circumstances outside the hospital may drift beyond your sphere of influence, and, despite visits from family and friends, you will feel uncomfortably cut off from the people and occasions that matter to you.

You have no choice in this: healing skin takes time, and there is little you can do but be patient. It is likely to be a very frustrating time: you lie there day by day, going through the hospital routine – punctuated by meals and cups of tea, probably without the energy or inclination to spend your time usefully. You lose your ability to concentrate on reading and find solace in listening to banal radio programmes, watching television mindlessly, or playing numerous card-games – Patience is a popular choice!

Some of the time you will mull over, and hopefully talk about, your facial damage and recovery with other patients or the staff. But many long-stay patients find themselves forced into a resigned state of flux and boredom that often verges on depression. Part of the reluctance and apprehension you may feel about frequent return visits to a plastic surgery unit – for, say, stays of three weeks – is due to the prior knowledge that you have of the conditions and of the psychological drawbacks you will experience.

And yet there is also a great security to be derived from a plastic surgery unit or other ward for the facially damaged. It is there that you can be totally accepted for what you are. Your fellow patients and the staff will not relate to you with any of the awkwardness or hostility you might meet outside. The hospital becomes, in effect, a second home, and one that it can be daunting to leave.

More importantly, you may well find that any affinity with members of the hospital staff is strictly restricted to the hospital confines. These are often relationships upon which you may depend considerably, and hospitalization would be miserable without them. Many different friends can be made – with staff from the highest to the lowliest – and they may constitute your first new friends made as a facially disfigured person. The friendships rarely survive beyond the end of your treatment, but they are none the slighter for that, especially if they are with the opposite sex.

Learning to be patient does not mean succumbing to morose passivity. You can be positively patient, but you will need help from all the various professional people involved in your treatment. For example, there would not appear to be much of a role for physiotherapists in your long-term facial reconstruction programme. But, while physios are helping you maintain your physical strength and keeping your limbs supple, they can perform the vital role of taking a regular enlightened interest in you and your well-being through your treatment: cajoling you when you are down, listening and advising as far as possible if the need arises, and giving another perspective on the slowness and progress of your treatment.

One of the worst aspects of long-term treatment is the inevitable surgical disappointment you will have to face. Surgery involves risks and sometimes expectations are not satisfied: a graft fails, infection takes hold, or some other setback interferes with your steady progress. My right eye proved to be particularly intractable, and I had to undergo several operations without making any significant improvement. In such circumstances the support of your family and friends is obviously valuable, but I found that someone outside my close circle was often able to provide the outlet for my impatience. To be a patient patient is well nigh impossible; if you bottle up your irritation, it is likely to fester and affect your will to keep going.

One particularly important hospital relationship is that between you and the medical team responsible for your treatment. The daily medical inspections that the junior medical staff undertake are valuable opportunities for you to ask questions and to develop an interest in your progress. The whole process of successfully changing faces will be that much easier if you do become involved in understanding your facial reconstruction.

There is a tendency among patients to become overawed in the presence of their surgeons and to slot into the category of 'Exhibit A'. You convince yourself that you should not speak unless spoken to, and that medical expertise is impossible to understand and won't be shared even if you ask. On both these counts I think you will be proved wrong, once you have broken the ice. I can well recall feeling like Exhibit A with no clothes on, as a crowd of medical students gathered around my bed to listen to a virtual lecture from my surgeon on my injuries and their treatment. At the end he coolly announced to his students that he would be away the next week, for he was attending a conference in Milan. I saw an opening: 'I won't be here next week either, I have a holiday booked in Rio de Janeiro'. My words seemed to come as a shock to the surgeon – a patient who could speak! This may seem an odd way to break the ice, but in a curious way my relationship with my rather socially awkward, if technically ingenious, surgeon changed for the better from that moment on. Other junior and senior doctors will respond in different ways, but the long journey of facial reconstruction will be that much more bearable if you feel less of a facial exhibit that is being moulded into shape and more of a personality involved in making decisions about your life in consultation with your surgical team.

The mysteries of medicine are beyond the layman's understanding: your ability to break out of the strait-jacket of the standard doctor–patient relationship will partly depend on your knowledge of some of the technical language. The subordinate social role that facially disfigured people tend to slip into – the feelings of inferiority and inadequacy – has to be challenged from an early stage for changing faces to be real and effective. If you assume you are at the mercy of surgical decisions and strategy, you will feel correspondingly powerless in life outside the hospital. Learning how to take an active part in your treatment gives you more confidence in the rest of your life.

It is not, of course, doctors who dominate the hospital scene. Facially injured people will soon realize the incredible debt they owe to the nursing staff for their unconditional and total support and sensitivity. Popular novels and soap operas do little for the image of nursing and often tend to miss the extraordinary dedication that you receive in the hospital bed. Some of the wounds, traumas and tragedies that nurses witness would leave ghastly emotional scars on lesser people; however, the depth of their training seems to give them a thicker skin and extra resilience.

Changing faces hinges more than anything on your confidence in being accepted as a personality, with your disfigurement as a part of that personality. Doctors, nurses and other hospital staff play a vital role in facial reconstruction and rehabilitation, a role that perhaps they are not always fully aware of. The success of your psychological recovery has its roots in the acceptance you receive in hospital: the journey of changing faces involves psychological as well as physical rebuilding, and everyone who comes into contact with you has a part to play.

CHAPTER 5

Classification of Burns and Surgical Treatment

Those who live and work in hospitals sometimes find it hard to see that they speak an almost foreign language. As a newly facially injured patient, you will be thrown into this medical world without the aid of a translator or dictionary. This can only be a cause of dismay, and, if you take no positive steps to remedy the situation, you can remain for weeks on end as an uninformed and ignorant recipient of hospital treatment.

Without knowledge of this language, you and your family are placed at an obvious disadvantage in communicating with medical and nursing staff. Although the medical and nursing professions are awakening to this fact, and a number of books do emphasize the importance of doctor–patient relationships, the ability of patients to pick up the hospital 'lingo' in the ward is still severely restricted. For example, the burns unit staff will use technical terms to describe your injuries or treatment. It may take you some time to figure out what they all mean, and even when you have discovered you may lack the confidence to use them in conversation. Some burns units have simple instruction sheets to translate the technicalities into layman's terms, and some plastic surgeons go out of their way to explain your problems clearly, but such help is by no means universal. Language training should be part of the treatment package in every burns unit along with feeding, bathing, bed-changing and drug dispensing.

There are reasons why it may be preferable from the point of view of the hospital staff to keep you in the dark in the early days. During the early 'shock' period it may be felt that you should not be given any cause for alarm, and that anyway you are too sick to be able to take in your position. However, for most patients with facial injuries there is just as much anxiety about injuries they are not told about as there is from the discovery of their actual extent. You can lie for some days knowing that you have severely injured your face but may be too terrified to ask for details: that is anxiety. To have the facts explained is often the first step to relieving some stress.

The earlier you can gain a working knowledge of the relevant medical vocabulary and a rudimentary understanding of your particular facial injury's medical details, the better. Without them, you can be no more than a passive observer of your facial reconstruction. With them, you can not only be a partner in decisions about your treatment but you can also appreciate, and start learning to live with, the limitations of the surgical (or other) techniques available.

The purpose of this chapter is to put words into your mouth – or the mouths of your relatives and friends – about your treatment and to help you understand your long-term prospects a little better. Because the technology of burns and plastic surgery changes so rapidly, only an outline will be provided here.

Classification of Burns

Skin burns are classified according to their depth.

Superficial burns involve damage only to the outer layer of the skin, typically after very short contact with a hot surface like an oven door. These wounds blister quickly and are red and very painful, but if allowed to dry out in sterile conditions will spontaneously heal and return to normal skin within a week to ten days.

Partial-thickness burns are deeper wounds that damage the nerve endings in the skin, thus making them extremely painful. This is the sort of burn that can result from a scald. They can heal naturally within two to three weeks. Thicker or the deeper partial-thickness (deep dermal) burns heal with greater difficulty and may require skin grafting.

Full-thickness burns completely destroy all skin layers, including sweat glands and hair follicles, and may even affect the subcutaneous tissues, for example, fat, muscle, tendon or bone. These wounds are the consequence of lengthy exposure to the very high temperatures caused by flames, some chemicals or electrical currents. They are the major focus of attention for the plastic surgeon because they do not heal. These deep open wounds are perfect sites for infection. Plastic surgeons are able to cover them with skin from other parts of your body (or from somebody else's in exceptional circumstances) – this is known as skin grafting. Grafting will not start until the surgeon judges that conditions are right.

The extent of your burns can be calculated by the 'Rule of Nine'. Your body is divided up into sections of 9 per cent of the total area: each arm is 9 per cent, each leg, 18 per cent, front and back trunk, 18 per cent, each, and the perineum 1 per cent. This surface area calculation of the burns also enables the doctors to work out the required fluid replacement. As well as the extent of your wounds other factors come into play – your age, your physical fitness, etc. In general, the younger and fitter the victim, the better he will be able to withstand the large fluid loss from the burned tissues. But the very young (under ten) are considered in the same way as older victims: for them any burn over 25 per cent is liable to be very serious indeed. Young, fit adolescents or adults stand a very good chance of surviving 40 per cent burns and two out of five can survive even if they suffer 70 per cent burns.

Once you are off the critical list, treatment for your wounds will be planned by your plastic surgeon. The basic outline of all post-burn treatment is, first, to create a 100 per cent skin cover; second, to attempt to rectify any major facial or other abnormalities; and, finally, to touch up and improve your tarnished facial looks.

The way each plastic surgeon approaches his subject for reconstruction very much depends on his training and his preferences. He has a wide range of 'tools' in his surgical kit-bag, from which he attempts to choose the most appropriate for the job in hand. No facially burned case will be treated the same as another – and different plastic surgeons have different ideas about best practice.

The first stage of facial reconstruction is really part of the overall programme to obtain 100 per cent skin replacement. If you have suffered extensive full-thickness burns, hospitalization may be lengthy. Skin grafts will be taken from your legs or other unaffected areas and used to cover all areas of unhealed partial- and full-thickness wounds.

Skin Grafts

Skin grafts can be classified according to their thickness and their ability to 'live' with their own blood supply.

Thin-split skin grafts are the simplest grafts available, being a very fine shaving of skin that is then laid on exposed, burned areas. These grafts are the main way of gaining 100 per cent skin cover. One advantage of these is that 'the donor site' (the area from which the graft is taken) heals rapidly. Within ten days donor sites return to normal and can be used again within weeks if the need arises. Donor sites are often far more painful than the deep injuries themselves, because the fine skimming of skin leaves all the nerve-ends in place and yelling.

The disadvantage of thin-split skin grafts is that they cannot withstand the contracting action of scars around their edges. As the scars tighten, which they tend to do, the grafts shrink too, and your facial symmetry will become distorted. Considerable efforts are made in burns units to prevent the contraction of scars. Pressure garments and facial masks may be used to prevent contractures of the grafted area, but these are not always successful.

Wolfe grafts are full-thickness grafts, small in dimension, and therefore able to 'take' like the thin-split skin grafts. They are more able to resist contraction and infection. They are not commonly used in the initial skin-replacement stage after burns, because the donor sites themselves will often require direct suture or thin-split skin grafts, which in their turn demand other suitable donor sites. In extensive burns cases, unaffected skin for donor sites is often in short supply and cannot be spared.

Full-thickness flaps are occasionally used in the early post-burn treatment of highly localized, deep burns, where structures such as tendons and joints are exposed.

There is sometimes a shortage of skin available for 'autografts', that is, grafts of your own skin. To make the most of what skin you can provide, long sheets of your skin are put through a 'meshing' machine to give them a kind of chicken-wire look and increase their spreadability by three or more times. The resulting grafted area is not particularly attractive, and thus this technique is rarely used on faces.

It is also possible to complement your own skin by using 'homografts' of skin from someone else. Skin can be stored in chilled conditions for several weeks and can be extremely valuable as a temporary skin cover for burn wounds, especially where the patient is not well enough to go through an operation to remove his own skin. Although you may 'reject' the skin eventually, while it provides cover it helps to prevent infection.

The success of any skin graft depends on a good blood supply in the recipient site: with an adequate supply, the new skin can adhere and become bonded within five days. If it has not done so in that time, it is unlikely that it ever will. The reasons for graft failure can be extremely frustrating: some blood clot or infection collected under the graft; the recipient site moved during the five days; or the recipient site was just unable to provide enough blood to enable the survival of the graft.

The Operation-dressing-operation Cycle

The process of patching up can stretch over some weeks. Your particular routine will be geared to regularly inspecting and dressing your burns. This routine is very variable and will differ from one burns unit to another. Your stamina to withstand this intensive treatment will be severely tested. A series of major operations in the space of a couple of months may be needed. Recovery from each of them may take a couple of days and you may well be immobilized for some spells in order to give your grafts the greatest chance of taking.

The dressing and inspection of grafts and the removal of donor-site bandages will be remembered as probably the least pleasant part of the patching up. You may be immersed in a warm saline bath to reduce the discomfort, but the risk of cross-infection often rules this out. Today burns units have, I'm glad to say, reduced the pain involved in the dressing procedure by employing new forms of analgesia/anaesthesia. This is a very skilled area and is still being perfected.

New anaesthetizing drugs have been developed (such as ketamine) that totally numb your senses but do not render you completely unconscious, and your breathing does not need assistance. You will be drowsy, but may be able to move a limb in a particular way when asked. Most importantly, you come round very quickly and with none of the after-effects of a general anaesthetic. Occasionally the drug will trigger hallucinatory images, but only in rare instances are these disturbing. Together with standard self-administered pain relief, these drugs have taken some of the worst pain and fear out of the operation-dressing-operation cycle.

During these weeks you will experience not only surgical treatment but also a programme of physiotherapy, occupational therapy and psychological assistance from the professionals associated with the burns unit. They will exercise your body and improve any lost co-ordination and concentration, try to iron out any psychological problems and generally prepare you for eventual discharge from hospital. If you have been seriously burned on your legs, it may be many weeks before you regain your feet, because all your leg grafts must be stable before you get upright again.

CHAPTER 6

Evaluating Plastic Surgery

All the king's horses and all the king's men,
Couldn't put Humpty together again.

As a facially disfigured person, plastic surgery is likely to be of considerable benefit to you. It aims to restore any part of the human anatomy that has been destroyed or maimed by disease or injury. The term 'plastic' derives from the Greek word meaning 'to mould', and plastic surgeons have developed a considerable armoury of techniques to mould improvements in people's appearance.

However, plastic surgery cannot magically re-create the natural good looks you have lost through injury or disease. These are lost for ever, and even the most skilled plastic surgeon cannot retrieve them. Changing faces involves coming to terms with that hard fact, although now, in the late-twentieth century, anyone disfigured can benefit from the massive strides taken by plastic surgery towards attaining perfection. Today's surgeons can transform and rebuild horribly ravaged faces and give them a presentability that even a few decades ago could not have been dreamed of. Recent developments in microsurgery technology hold out hope for further improvements in the years to come.

You can be confident, then, that the distorted and scarred mess of a face that you see in the mirror need not remain as a hideous mask for the rest of your life. With perseverance and some luck, you can recover a facial appearance that, though still 'different', has some semblance of normality.

How Much Plastic Surgery Should be Done?

At the start of your treatment, and at many times during it, you will have to take stock of what the future holds and ask yourself, 'Is more surgery required?' It sometimes surprises people that such a query could arise: surely you must have 'a full course'? Plastic surgery can go on and on making improvements to a disfigured face, but, as this book aims to show, changing faces involves a change in one's self-belief, attitudes and face values. There is a lot more to changing faces than undergoing plastic surgery.

I was asked only recently when I was next 'going in' for surgery, and was met with astonishment when I replied that I haven't had any surgery for fifteen years and don't intend having any more. Similarly, in a job interview I was once asked if I thought I needed more plastic surgery, to which I rather brashly replied, 'Do you think I need more?' You should be aware that in the public mind there is the unwritten assumption that facial oddities and marks can be completely removed with sufficient plastic surgery. The reality is that surgery can remove and replace the worst blemishes but is unable to re-create or conjure up your lost natural looks.

It is worth quoting a couple of plastic surgeons to bear out this point. The first, Sir Archibald McIndoe – to many the founding father of modern plastic surgery – said in the late 1940s after he had done considerable work with burned fighter pilots: 'It is not possible to construct a face of which the observer is unconscious, but it should not leave in his mind an impression of revulsion, and the patient himself should not be an object of remark or pity.' A well-known American plastic surgeon of more recent times, Richard Stark,* has written: 'Although my (surgical) results have not succeeded in making the patients look exactly as they did before their trauma, their appearance no longer repels or evokes pity. A completely aesthetic result is a tall order. For the patient it becomes a crusade; for the surgeon, a solemn contract.'

How far the pursuit of facial perfection becomes 'a crusade' for you will depend on your answers to a series of questions. The issues raised by these questions require very careful consideration: you must take time to talk out the problems with those close to you and with anyone else whose judgement you respect. On some questions you will need the professional guidance of

* R. B. Stark, *Total Facial Reconstruction* (Gower, 1984).

your plastic surgeon with whom you need to strike up a communicative relationship.

Your facial reconstruction may seem to be your problem only. It isn't. You will benefit by hearing other people's perspectives, and, at the same time, they will benefit from being open with you about their thoughts and opinions. Changing faces is not something you will go through in isolation from the rest of humanity: facial disfigurement is, above all, a social handicap, and your course of surgery to try to diminish it must at least partially respect the wishes of the wider society in which you will circulate. This may suggest that you have to fulfil certain minimum social standards when deciding on how much plastic surgery to receive – and these are not easily discovered. Talking to others will help you to do so.

It would be impossible for this book, indeed, any book, to give you the answer to the question of how much plastic surgery to have, but I think you can best tackle it by pondering a set of interrelated questions:

How much does facial perfection matter to you?

What can plastic surgeons offer to improve your looks?

What sacrifices will you have to make to have the surgery?

The Matter of Facial Perfection

Since so much seems to hinge on having good looks in today's culture, you may be tempted to say that it is absolutely imperative that you do everything you can to better and improve your disfigured face. Indeed, you may argue that you would be thought stupid and rather thoughtless if you did not go as far as you could with surgery. On the other hand, you could argue that it is pure vanity and needless self-indulgence to concentrate on your tarnished face. People, you may think, should take you as they find you – appearances are deceptive, aren't they?

Both these opposing viewpoints recognize the social significance we all attach to our faces. They are the most obvious outward canvas upon which we can display our personality. It is, of course, true that even the most disfigured face can convey something of the personality behind it, but your opportunity to do this may be seriously restricted by the fact that your severe disfigurement may make it more difficult for other people to approach you. Your face will not attract but may repel attention, and social acceptance may therefore be that much harder to obtain. Your face is obviously important to you personally too. Irrespective of your social circumstances, your assessment of yourself, your self-respect and self-confidence are bound to be tied up with your facial looks. We are all, to some extent, conscious of cultural forces like the advertising industry, which tell us what we ought to aspire to look like, and how wonderful we would feel if we looked 'better'. But quite apart from these, any departure from your 'normal' reflection in the mirror is bound to be disturbing. A disfiguring accident will therefore initially leave you out of joint with respect to your face. It is not just women who tend to be particularly demoralized by the loss of facial symmetry; men too pride themselves on their appearance and are prepared to spend considerable sums to make it more 'appealing', because 'attractiveness' is apparently so very dependent on facial looks.

The common immediate response to disfigurement tends to be a desire to recapture your past visage – your crusade has started. For some this is the start of a lifelong quest for perfection: they are willing to undergo any number of surgical procedures to 'fine tune' their new face. Unfortunately, they may become so obsessed with this that they fail to make any meaningful effort to rebuild their lives. Their surgical repair supersedes their social rehabilitation and makes that transition impossibly difficult. In effect, these people get stuck in the belief that until they have cleansed their face, they stand no social chance whatever.

This sort of psychological trap can be even more enveloping once the disfigured person discovers the mammoth time commitment required for a succession of surgical operations. Plastic surgery is a long-term treatment process that cannot be unduly hurried. For someone who prizes facial appearance very highly, this technical slowness can be frustrating and yet can justify self-isolation. Their retreat from social contact can be reinforced by their presumption that until they are facially restored, they will not find any social acceptability, won't make friends and will be cold-shouldered.

At the other extreme from these 'perfectionists' are those

disfigured people who seem almost to revel in their tarnished looks and show reluctance to go through surgical reconstruction. They use their disfigurement as an excuse for other social failings such as their inability to get a job. They may become very embittered about the treatment given to disfigured people and determined not to 'give in' by improving their facial looks. For this sort of person, the crusade is not for their own facial renovation but rather for a change in social attitudes to the disfigured in particular and the handicapped in general.

I have deliberately contrasted the two extreme reactions to disfigurement and approaches to plastic surgery because most disfigured people will have experienced both extremes – the search for perfection or the refusal to undergo more surgery – at different times in their journey of changing faces. I can certainly recall times when I have yearned for a better face and others when I have used my face as a justification for feeling bitter about my plight.

There are unquestionably minimum social standards of facial acceptability to which it is important the disfigured conform, but you may find it difficult to decide what they are. A few years after my accident, still looking very badly disfigured, I travelled to India. There, and in Iran and Afghanistan, my face was rarely given the slightest attention. Heavily scarred faces are regular sights, as disfiguring diseases and accidents are commonplace, while plastic surgery is not widely available in these countries. I could quite easily have lived and worked there with no further surgery. But on my return, a trip on the London Underground was enough to convince me that I needed more reconstruction to live and work in Britain.

Once you have satisfied the minimum standards, should you then continue to seek improvements? You have to compare the benefits of further facial advances with the costs on your time and lifestyle of doing so, and then make that judgement for yourself. Such a comparison can be successfully conducted only with the help and advice of the professional staff responsible for your treatment.

The Plastic Surgeon's Repertoire

Discovering a realistic view of your facial possibilities will not be as straightforward as it sounds. You may expect your surgeon to look at you at the start of your plastic surgery and predict the finished product. Very few surgeons are prepared to commit themselves in such a way, partly because they are unwilling to raise false hopes and expectations. They may also prefer a cautious approach, because their plans for you may change and develop as your surgery progresses.

More importantly, however, your ability to appreciate their technical ideas may well be very limited – mine was – and it may take you some years to learn the language that allows you to communicate with the head of your surgical team. You may find it easier to gain some indication of your future prospects by picking the brains of experienced nurses or physiotherapists. Their day-to-day contact with you may give you the confidence to raise very crucial questions. 'What are my chances?' 'Will I ever look the same again?' 'What is ahead of me?'

The darkness that some disfigured people live in as regards the possibilities of plastic surgery is almost total. They are given some vague ideas about their next operation, told to turn up on a certain day, sign the consent form and undergo the surgery with no complaints. This is often not the fault of the surgeon, who may have tried in his own way to explain the details of his facial strategy, but is simply a consequence of the patient's unfamiliarity with the descriptive terms used.

Some plastic surgery units go to great lengths to describe the various procedures to their patients, for example by using simple diagrammatic sheets. There is undoubtedly a greater willingness today than there was a decade ago to share the technical possibilities with patients, and yet, ironically, the technology of plastic surgery has become increasingly sophisticated and unintelligible to the layman.

The language of microsurgery, now a powerful technique in plastic surgery, may need detailed translation – even nurses and other professionals can find communication on such technical details difficult. Furthermore, understanding one surgical technique of today may be of little help to you tomorrow when a new innovation becomes available. The speed of technological advance has quickened in the past decade. The recently appointed first professor of plastic surgery in Britain, Gus McGrouther, wants to see an acceleration in worldwide research to extend the specialty's range of techniques still further.*

Plastic Surgery Techniques – A Bit of History

The history of facial reconstructive surgery has its roots in the work of several pioneers during and after the First World War, although there had been some early attempts to recover a few facially injured people's looks in the aftermath of the American Civil War in the 1860s. The numerous blast injuries and shrapnel wounds of soldiers, sailors and airmen during the First World War accelerated the search for effective techniques of facial reconstruction.

Sir Harold Gillies was given the job by the government of the day of developing better methods, and all patients needing such operations were directed to him at a single hospital, Queen's Hospital in Sidcup, Kent. There, over many years, he and his team specialized in, and perfected, several new options, notably by using full-thickness skin grafts, including pedicle flaps (now seldom used).

In England the Second World War gave further impetus to this new surgical speciality, and four surgeons in hospitals in St Albans, Stoke Mandeville, Basingstoke and East Grinstead made major advances. Sir Archibald McIndoe at East Grinstead operated on over 3,500 RAF pilots and aircrew, many of whom displayed the classic 'airman's burns' of severe wounds to eyelids, nose, cheeks, lips and chin. He preferred to use a combination of partial-thickness grafts and pedicle flaps.

His most memorable contribution to plastic surgery – and perhaps to medicine as a whole – was his foundation of the Guinea Pig Club for men who went through the East Grinstead experience. He realized that not even the most brilliant surgery could, by itself, rehabilitate the facially injured. The rebuilding of shattered lives had to take place alongside the facial reconstruction, and the Club was one sign of this. But he also made a point of developing a long-term surgical plan for, and with, each

* *Guardian*, 19 April 1989.

patient, and this usually meant very lengthy hospitalization and many operations – up to fifty in some cases.

By the 1950s the skills of plastic surgeons were starting to leap into uncharted territory. Up until then most facial surgery had involved the use of skin grafts from different parts of the body, with the result that a rather motley and patchwork-quilt effect was produced. The colours of the different skin grafts would not necessarily tie in well. This prompted surgeons to make increasing use of large skin flaps. There is now, with the use of microsurgical techniques, a good chance that these skin flaps can be quickly and effectively used to create very smooth, single-colour and aesthetically acceptable facial looks.

Microsurgery

The most advanced plastic surgery is now capable of extensive facial reconstruction. These major procedures are rarely attempted until at least a year after injury, but, when all is ready, the surgeon and his team may plan a whole series to be completed in quite a short time, like a year, followed up perhaps by a few extra 'touch-up' operations later on.

These facial reconstructions commonly employ a mixture of sizeable partial-thickness grafts and large skin flaps that allow burned or scarred tissues to be removed and replaced with smooth, unblemished skin of a matching colour. The very careful choice of where the edges of these flaps and grafts will finish can greatly improve the aesthetic effect, because the edges can be skilfully blended into the facial contours. Another advantage of these flaps and grafts over the skin-cover techniques of the burns surgeon is that by using thicker layers of skin, the scars do not contract at all once in place.

Microsurgery has given the plastic surgeon an extra dimension to his skill. The use of an operating microscope has greatly reduced the time and risk in flap surgery. The surgeon can now take a full-thickness skin flap from one place and in one step 'knit' it on to the intended recipient site. The blood vessels in the two can be literally joined up together with the help of fine surgical methods.

The art of flap surgery is moving ahead every year. Several

living examples of total facial reconstruction after horrible facial injuries or disease can testify to that. The great bonus of microsurgery is the speed at which facial improvements can be made. Some surgeons now attempt to compress several major facial operations into perhaps a month, working on the premise that as long as the patient is fit, long delays are unnecessary and may be detrimental to his morale. Problems can arise in any operation or plan – a little infection, a poor 'take', a slow recovery from an operation. But these are risks that the surgeon and the patient must take.

Although dramatic improvements in facial reconstructions have been possible in recent years, do not imagine that microsurgery can completely remove disfigurement. Disfigurement is only diminished, not overcome. The public is often led to believe in the miraculous powers of plastic surgery: articles appear in fashion magazines or newspapers that make claims like this: 'It is a startling fact that you no longer have to put up with any part of yourself that you don't like. In theory you can be virtually remodelled to your specification.'* Although this particular article did admit that 'there is still no absolute way to make scars disappear altogether', the impression given is that plastic surgery can work miracles.

Unfortunately, once you have been facially injured or impaired, you cannot be surgically restored. But you can now enjoy the skills and experience of plastic surgeons who have tested and refined their procedures on facially injured people over the last half-century and more.

Making Sacrifices for Surgery

The Guinea Pigs of McIndoe's surgery often went through fifty or more major operations during their facial reconstruction. Today's surgery is quicker, less risky and more aesthetically effective. But it is not done without imposing considerable strains on you, the patient, and your family. This is particularly true for disfigured children, who may, as they grow, have to return for further corrective operations. But for adults too plastic surgery is still a

---

* 'Body Sculpture', *Good Housekeeping*, July 1988.

long drawn-out course of treatment that lasts several years in most cases. For although microsurgery has reduced the time factor in most skin-flap transfers, many plastic surgeons are unwilling to operate again until the skin has settled down, perhaps a time of six months.

Your willingness to go back for more operations may well flag, as you gradually rehabilitate yourself outside and as you increasingly balance the extra facial benefits to be derived from the next operation against the costs. It is a good idea for you to agree some kind of plan with your surgeon, whereby you commit yourself to a phase of operations, after which you take stock before confirming that you will undergo the next phase. This will allow you to assess your facial gains frequently and identify your next preferred improvements. It also has the added advantage of letting your surgeon appreciate that you have a controlling role in the surgery.

You are the one who must make the ultimate decision as to whether to go ahead or not. You are the one who will suffer the discomfort and pain – and, despite adequate analgesia and highly sensitive nursing, these are ever present. You are the one who has to face the anticipation and fear of needles and operations. You are the one who may have to leave your family in difficult circumstances or put your job in jeopardy. You are the one who has to endure hospitalization, the loss of freedom and privacy, and you are the one who could be choosing to spend your time in many more enjoyable ways than in an operating theatre. You hold the reins!

The impact of facial disfigurement can be greatly diminished by a course of surgery. You will have to draw on considerable reserves of stamina and even courage to stay the course, but the benefits of doing so are that your friends and family and the public in general will not be appalled by your face or, hopefully, embarrassed to be seen with you.

In conjunction with the surgeon, you must choose how much surgery to have. Although a certain minimum amount will be essential, changing faces is a process in which, despite your disfigurement, you have to gain the confidence to let your personality shine through and overshadow the physical features of your face. Plastic surgery will help you to feel a new person, but it will not make you one.

PART 2

Reconstructing Your Life

CHAPTER 7

Taking up the Challenge of Disfigurement

The physical improvement in your facial appearance that can be achieved by a course of plastic surgery will not in itself be enough to enable you to change faces, to live a full and enjoyable life again. Whether you have suffered facial damage from birth, or been injured later in life, operations on your physical imperfections are only part of living with your facial difference. Along with the exterior transformation must inevitably go internal, psychological changes.

At first, your reactions to your new face may be dispiriting – I discussed them briefly in Chapter 1. As time passes and you live with your new face, these early feelings may harden and make your further recovery more complicated. Even though you may be gradually seeing your face transformed through surgical interventions, your psychological progress may be slow and hesitating.

This chapter looks at how your disfigurement will hit you psychologically. The process of changing faces requires that you fully realize your disfigurement and be realistic about what it means for you. This realization does not come from sitting in front of a mirror, staring at yourself – that will only help to prove that you do have an odd-looking face.

What I mean by 'realizing' is a much more profound appreciation of your new life prospects, not in an emotional and perhaps frustrated way, but honestly and soberly.

Being Disfigured

Your first looks in the mirror may have given you a nasty shock. You may have spent some days or weeks in suspended belief – 'Can this really have happened to me?' When the truth of your injuries does start to sink in, you may still believe that they will be only temporary and that in a couple of months' time, you will be able to regain your lost looks and take up your life again where you left off.

How long you persist in this sort of thinking will depend on whether your close friends or the hospital staff treating you are prepared to shatter your illusions. They may be worried about doing so and may well allow you to go on pretending. Sooner or later, though, you will have to acknowledge that things will never be the same again – you are disfigured for life.

What does this mean? Disfigurement has two dimensions: I shall call them the personal and the social dimensions. They indicate the change that you have to go through in becoming disfigured, and how you are seen by others.

Personal disfigurement refers to the change that takes place in your perception of yourself. The sort of mental picture you have of yourself and your body will be radically altered. Although you may possess the same eyes for seeing, voice for talking and mind for thinking, you will alter the way you think of your face.

It is not just your body-image that will change but also the way you conduct and speak about yourself. If you have been previously 'normal-faced', you will have adopted mannerisms and habits of mind that have evolved since your early childhood. Your looks, your body language and your spoken attitudes were previously reliable guides to your character. In their place you now have a disfigured face and, as a result, massive uncertainty about how to relate to others. In effect, your personal evaluation of your own worth may well be threatened: it will be hard for you to maintain your self-respect because your face is now so blemished and battered.

Social disfigurement is the way in which your disfigurement will be viewed in the eyes of others. Your facial oddities will now mark you out as different, and you will, without any choice, join the ranks of the 'handicapped' in society. What this means is that you now have a very conspicuous and, as seen in the eyes of others, debilitating trait that makes it difficult for them to behave normally with you. They may bring assumptions about 'the disfigured' as a whole to bear when deciding how best to behave with you.

Reactions to Realizing Your Disfigurement

For many victims, the moment of realization of their disfigurement is often a crisis point when something clicks and the full spotlight shines on their predicament. For me, it was a first visit to a pub with an old friend – I sat and suddenly felt my disfigurement in all its fullness, as people either stared or asked curious questions like 'What happened to him?'

The moment of truth can seriously interrupt what had been a smooth process of recovery. You may have been living in hope. Now your eyes are opened. When you first look at your face, you are shocked by your new physical looks; you may react angrily, defeatedly, miserably, stoically or otherwise. You need to be able to express your emotion and devastation and talk it out so that you are prepared to put up with all the discomfort and hospitalization that you will need to go through to have your face physically rebuilt.

Realizing the permanence of your disfigurement, however, may take place several months after you have first looked at yourself. You will probably have been discharged from hospital and may be trying to start up your life again, when suddenly you perceive the hugeness of the hurdles that you have to face and overcome. You will have probably lost some of the hospital support system that was such a wonderful cocoon. Now you are out in the world, isolated, and your eyes are no longer glazed with hope. Your disfigurement is obvious and you are experiencing it, hourly, daily.

Disfigured people react in different ways to these circumstances. A combination of low reactions is perfectly natural – and, indeed, in changing faces you have to go through some very negative phases during which the world and your prospects have little to commend them. What is worrying is if any of them take complete hold over you and last for a long period. If this is the case, don't just wallow in your negativity; get help from someone trained and skilled in helping.

Denial. You may still refuse to accept your new situation, or admit it only in your 'best' moods. This is a sensible self-protection technique and may well allow you to exist in social isolation but will be difficult to sustain in public.

Anxiety. You become very nervous and agitated at going anywhere for fear of being exposed to the sort of horrors you imagine people like you are bound to meet. You become a 'worrier', someone who is never at ease, never relaxed and never able to talk naturally about their feelings.

Depression. You lose your drive and zest for life and become extremely despondent about yourself and your life. You may look for ways of relieving your low spirits – perhaps alcohol or antidepressant drugs – but they may have the reverse effect and dependence on them may increase.

These very common reactions to disfigurement are often seen in various sorts of behaviour that are symptomatic of the shock of your sudden discovery. You may adopt an almost child-like dependence on your family; you may become highly self-centred and unable to acknowledge other people's needs and worries; you may withdraw completely from contact with other people; you may seek to blame other people for your own inadequacies; you may try to buy your way into new circles of friends with expensive purchases or over-elaborate gestures.

Your inner struggle at this stage may be focused on your strange half-way position in terms of being handicapped. Someone with facial disfigurement isn't handicapped in the same way as a person in a wheelchair, for example. And yet as a disfigured person you are socially handicapped because of your odd-looking face. You may be very uncertain which side of the fence to come down on: you will be tempted to identify with the handicapped and thereby accept the norms and expectations attached to being handicapped – less social achievement possible, lower social status expected, a dependent person and so on. On the other hand, your previous normal-faced existence will still attract you, but you are aware that you may not be able to live with the standards and expectations of your former peer groups. You fear that if you do try to be part of normal society, you may 'fail' by your earlier criteria. Your inadequacy may turn into inferiority.

You are at a crossroads: in one direction lies a life of less stress but one of less excitement; in the other, the one that I hope you will choose, lies a life full of challenges, and pitfalls too. To take it, to decide to take on your face and live a full life by 'normal society' standards is difficult, but it can be done. The rest of the book is intended to help you to do it.

Re-entry into the Public Eye

Rather like the American Space Shuttle, you need to have an extra-thick layer of protection for re-entry into your 'atmosphere'. Special tiles protect the Shuttle from the heat of burn-up on re-entry. Your extra-tough layer has to be capable of withstanding and deflecting not physical heat but rather the withering attention of other people. Unfortunately, the extra layer does not just miraculously appear: you have to construct it, probably with considerable help from others.

As you start to 'go public', two interrelated feelings are likely to dominate your thinking.

1. You feel very noticeable. Everyone is bound to look at you, but, instead of their glances passing on to other people or events, your face sticks out and interferes with their normal behaviour and assumptions about you as a fellow human being. You will be aware of how noticeable you are. Most people aren't used to being inspected, being in the firing line, and in the past you probably ensured that you didn't stand out too much – low profiles are more comfortable.

2. You will be hypersensitive to any action, word or gesture that you can interpret as indicative of other people's reactions to you. You may completely misjudge some reactions by reading too much into them. This is particularly likely if you have already predicted what sort of reaction you expect to receive, because you start looking to confirm those predictions. For example, if you forecast that you will be thought of as 'a bit thick', you will assume that anybody who shows signs of reluctance to talk to you is thinking that you are half-witted, when actually their reticence may just be because they are confused and unsure of themselves.

The main message of this part of the book is really that the way in which you conduct yourself on re-entry will critically affect how you are received. 'Do as you would be done by' sums it up –

if you are positive, the world will take you positively. But if you are downcast, the natural sympathy that people may feel for you will probably be less forthcoming. Looking depressed is unlikely to gain you much sympathy. Try and be open and honest, and people will find it easier to express their real concern for you – and help you to see that they acknowledge you as a whole and worthwhile person.

So here's the contradiction: you have to toughen yourself for the trials of re-entry but not in a defensive, armour-plated way. Your armour comes from being willing to be open, thereby deflecting and parrying all curiosity or hostility. In effect, you should aim to understand other people's initial reactions and build on them so that you direct them to your advantage.

On its own, this type of 'reactive' behaviour will not be enough. In some situations you cannot afford to wait for people to react and then devise your own response. You have also to be 'pro-active', which means displaying yourself actively rather than passively. You have to be prepared to take the initiative. Because of their ignorance about the causes of facial disfigurement, people you meet may assume you are suspicious or mentally retarded, or they may try to patronize you and treat you as a poor unfortunate. It is important you squash their misconceptions and assert your worth.

You may be surprised at how little people know about facial impairment. Many people probably suspect that you might have been in a fire or have undergone a major cancer operation, but there will be considerable uncertainty about how to approach you, just in case they have got it all wrong. In such circumstances, if you merely react passively, you may make these nervous people even more uneasy. It may be much better to lay your cards on the table – 'Yes, I was burned, but I'm OK' – just a few simple words to get the subject into the open. By taking the initiative, you put them at ease.

A pro-active approach that offers information will enable you to communicate more easily, but each situation has to be weighed up and assessed. You must develop acute antennae for responding to any given meeting. Being very aware of what is happening around you will help you to select an appropriate tactic. It gets easier for you as you become more familiar with other people's initial reactions, but it is always the first time for them. You won't get it right first time or every time. Trial and error will be required – and so will a good deal of bravery. Sometimes trying out a new ploy may seem almost foolhardy, but if it achieves your aim of being treated normally, or at least not as an idiot, it will have done the trick. For example, I find it hard to imagine myself doing the following, recalled by my brother: 'I remember going with you to pubs and being aware of conversations stopping and eyes drilling into our backs. In one, you completely disarmed a group of starers with the throwaway comment, "Not looking at my best today, I'm afraid."'

There are a number of general responses that, as a disfigured person, you are likely to come across. I've called the group of them the SCARED syndrome – Staring, Curiosity, Anguish, Recoil, Embarrassment and Dread – and have devoted the whole of Chapter 10 to discussing how you can handle each one. So frequently will you come across them that you will become almost expert at framing your own particular way of communicating yourself. Remember too that you are far more familiar with facing awkward moments than are the people you meet. This should give you the confidence to adopt pro-active means of communicating.

I am well aware how very difficult it is for some disfigured people to be outgoing. Their personalities just do not seem to lend themselves to being forceful, and they will not thrive on their new noticeabililty. They are naturally reserved. My tactical suggestions might seem to have only limited relevance for them. But I think changing faces does change us all (the disfigured and those they meet) in different ways, and one thing is certain: you cannot rely on face-value judgements any more.

Your attitude to the world has to become more extrovert, so as to convey the message that you are really all right. You might be even more interesting to know because of your disfigurement . . . Natural reserve was OK before, but it won't bring you much reward now. So take the plunge – what have you got to lose?

CHAPTER 8

Rebuilding Self-esteem

Rebuilding shattered lives is no easy matter, and there are no miracle cures, but it is possible. What I shall try to do in this chapter is outline some of the attitudes of mind that can play a part in successful facial recovery. The combination of messages that will be most relevant to *you* is impossible for me to judge, although my hope is that I will strike a few chords that might lead you through a difficult patch in your rehabilitation.

Changing faces is an on-going process, and what might boost self-esteem today may make you feel depressed tomorrow. Rebuilding calls for more than one-day-wonder boosts. Your will to swim through some very low moods and to resist the continual temptation to cut yourself off from the rest of the world will be sorely tested at times.

You are likely to place great demands on the love and energies of your family and close friends. They may be your only source of positive messages of encouragement. You may also gain solace from hospital staff, social workers and psychotherapists, all of whom can help to rebuild your self-esteem. Groups of like-minded, similarly afflicted people (self-help groups or others in your hospital ward) may help to bolster your self-respect, as you learn from others of their problems and achievements. In Chapter 9 I have looked at the role of all these important people, but here I want to concentrate on your individual feelings and thought processes.

You are Not a Write-off

All facially injured people fear that the loss of their physical attractiveness will definitely reduce their likeability. They imagine that facial disfigurement is so off-putting to those whom they meet, or would like to communicate with, that their chances of meaningful socializing are greatly reduced. You are not alone in this anxiety. In fact, you join the ranks of many of the handicapped groups in society, who feel that they have sunk to the status of second-class citizens.

You may be well aware that the link between normal physical good looks and likeability seems very firmly fixed in today's collective consciousness, and many cultural forces serve only to underline it. Advertisements, for example, tend to stress the benefits of beauty and cosmetic purity – you can see this in the pages of any women's magazine. Most of us grow up with fairytales reinforcing the strong impression that misshapen bodies and ugly faces contain mean and unpleasant personalities. This sort of association has gone so far that even normal-faced women can be trapped by an obsession to attain real physical beauty, failing in the process to see that their normal, if rather plain, face is only a part of what makes them a whole person – their kindness, sensitivity, wit, charm or other attributes are all undervalued in their obsessional search for beauty.

So you aren't the only one who feels 'written-off' because of your looks. But you may feel more of a 'write-off' than the normal-faced physically disabled person or the person who is obsessed with his inadequate looks. Your looks have been completely ruined, and you no longer have the smooth complexion and symmetrical features that for years you took for granted.

What you have actually lost in being disfigured are two social advantages. First, you have lost the chance of being automatically accepted into any social gathering as just an ordinary person. You will always be noticeable and will feel continually 'on trial'. Any natural human faults or failings on your part are, you think, going to count against you. Thus, you will become far more conscious of your weaknesses than your good points. Your self-confidence tends to evaporate and you write yourself off – quite unnecessarily. Secondly, your facial damage brings you much unwanted attention. You stick out in crowds; you are noticeable wherever you go. If you fail to give convincing 'answers' to this public inquisition, you fear that people will interpret this as further evidence that your facial disfigurement conceals a low-value personality. Again, by letting yourself think you have failed in public, you condemn yourself to being a 'write-off'.

In a similar way, you may feel that your previous friends won't be interested in knowing you now, because they won't want to be seen with you for fear that they too will be labelled 'odd'. However, you will probably be surprised at how your friends – your good, close friends – actually take you completely as you are with no scruples or write-off attitudes. If one or two of them do adopt hostile postures, you are best rid of them.

Or again, you may feel written-off as regards making new friends. Sometimes it is not easy to break the ice, this is true. But once you have, you will open up unexpected depths of friendship and warmth. Friendships and relationships do not depend on facial perfection. In fact, in my experience my disfigurement has probably helped me to make friends rather than inhibited me, because you really get to know someone quickly once you start having a frank conversation about facial disfigurement!

If you are young and single, you may fear that facial disfigurement will consign you to the group of unloved outcasts who will never again share good times with the opposite sex. Here again you are falling into the 'beauty trap' where physical beauty is seen as a necessary precondition for happiness, especially in marriage. But if there is one thing that TV soap operas do truthfully illustrate, it is that wealth and beauty are no guarantee of happiness. We all know this intuitively anyway, but we have been conditioned to the contrary over the years by all those advertisements.

To write yourself off as a potential partner in a meaningful relationship is to give credence to the myth that good looks are a prerequisite to good relationships. 'Normal'-faced people don't automatically find the right partner; some never do. You, as a disfigured person, stand just as good a chance as they do, assuming you don't cut yourself off from social contact. And what is more, you may well find that your ability to have an honest and adult relationship is actually improved by your disfigurement. Certainly there will be no illusions about being loved for your looks alone!

So don't write yourself off. The arguments I have put forward here are some that you could bring to bear when you do feel in a negative mood. But you will soon come to realize that these self-denigrating attitudes are not quickly shifted unless more positive ones are available to take their place.

Be Realistic about Your Future

The sort of logic that sometimes afflicts the facially disfigured goes something like this: 'I've never seen anyone looking like me doing anything useful in public; all such deformed people must be hiding away, having lost all faith in themselves; I can't see any point in trying to do anything, because I know I'll be rejected, just like them, so I might as well hide too.'

You'll lose the changing faces battle before you start if you think like that. Admittedly, there is a view held by a few people that disfigured people can't make much of a contribution, can't look after themselves; they look suspicious and don't have many friends. This is the myth that anyone and everyone who is disfigured can – and must – refute utterly, because, if anything, you will be more able to do many things – useful things – being disfigured than not. What you have been through and suffered is likely to make you a more compassionate and caring person, at the very least.

In rebuilding self-esteem, one thing to your advantage is that the pressure to succeed – whatever that might mean – has been lifted as a result of your disfigurement. Your family and your peers will probably reassess your prospects downwards: their ambitions for you will be lowered. But *you* need not lower your ambitions. They may have to be redirected, but as long as your mind and body are still alive – even if disfigured – you stand a chance.

The redirection of your life and your criteria of what constitutes 'success' will take time to evolve. There is no reason why you should achieve less than you had intended, although *what* you achieve may be different. For example, if your ambition had been to rise up the ladder in a company, union or profession, you may gradually find your vision altering to take account of your new circumstances – perhaps you think it will now be impossible for you to be a high-profile leadership figure, or you may even feel that those goals are less worthwhile than you once thought and that now you would prefer to get involved in social or charity work. A change of tack like this will not mean you achieve less; you have just set yourself different goals.

In judging what your life is worth, you will have to take your disfigurement into account. You will see that some activities are more or less barred to you because of your disfigurement, especially, for example, jobs in the public eye. But other doors will open up. You may not be able to go on the stage with your disfigurement, but you will be able to empathize with the plight of minority groups of one sort or another in a way you could never do before. You may find immense satisfaction from totally new areas of work.

An important distinction can be made here. It is sometimes suggested that you, the disfigured, have got to adjust to your new (unfortunate) situation – it's tragic, but you'll just have to adapt your lifestyle and expectations accordingly, i.e., downwards. Merely adjusting in this way, however, will not help you build up your self-esteem again, because you will be passively accepting other people's views of what disfigured people can – or ought not to be allowed to – do.

You must start to see your circumstances as no more than the base camp from which your future life begins. It is up to you to make meaningful decisions: you can walk with, talk with, love with, compete with, shop with, drink with, do all sorts of things with others, even though you are disfigured. So do not be bound by what you think others think (or what you might think) disfigured people are limited to doing. Within reason, you can do anything!

See It as a Challenge

Demoralization and disfigurement often go hand in hand. A disfigured person who has lost confidence in himself and who has little or no support from other people will probably seek out fellow sufferers who are similarly alienated. Their stories of social disasters, feelings of rejection and lack of any strategy to improve their situation make it even harder to start getting to grips with facial disfigurement as a positive challenge.

Your disfigurement will undoubtedly make enormous demands on you (and your family), and you may not believe in the early days that you have either the ability or the stamina to stay the course. You may feel the prospect of living with facial scars and deformity is beyond you. None the less, if you can see your way to viewing your future as unpredictable but interesting, you may realize what I mean by a challenge.

For me, the motivation for the challenge came initially from understanding how close to death I had been and how glad I was to be alive – even though disfigured. It also comes from a desire to live the rest of my life to the full – I couldn't bear the idea of missing out on life. My facial injuries gave, if anything, an added dimension to my life, making my future even more intriguing than it had been before. Could I really do anything with a ruined face? It was a challenge to find out. And in finding out that the answer was definitely yes, my self-confidence returned – and as arrogantly as before!

This sounds as if the challenge is a purely self-centred affair. In fact, the biggest challenge is to learn to handle public situations of all sorts. Whereas in childhood you automatically and unselfconsciously learn how to communicate with, and relate to, your friends, family and the world in general, the process of changing faces is an acutely self-conscious process of resocialization. You have to redevelop much of your social behaviour in the face of unremitting public attention and much curiosity. If you set about this resocialization reluctantly or with resentment, you may well fail to adopt the appropriate communication skills. As will be stressed in later chapters, the people you meet may need you to help them to reconsider their preconceived and possibly awkward reactions to you. You will also need to perfect non-verbal communication skills to reassure those people whom you can't speak to of your normality.

One popular view of disfigured individuals is that they are difficult to have a conversation with, because it is so painful to look them in the face. You therefore have to break down this barrier if you want to start communicating – and when you succeed, you will challenge them too. Not only will they discover their misconception about you, but they will also have their eyes opened as regards disabled or handicapped people. Nobody will want to communicate with you if you wear your new face with dismay and sadness.

Seeing your facial damage as a challenge is quite the opposite to seeing it as a complete, life-time personal disaster. There are many wonderful examples of men and women overcoming handicaps in positive and extravagant ways. If asked, almost all would say, I think, that their disability was a spur to perfection or betterment rather than a dampener on it. They refuse to be categorized as disabled or handicapped and thereby given special treatment or excuses for any inadequacies in social communication. Instead they shake off their physical limitations and confound everyone by their feats and achievements. Their infectious enthusiasm points the way for so many of us, even if we do not possess their extrovert, even belligerent, personalities. Anyone trying to come to terms with facial disfigurement has to be prepared to change the emphasis of his personality. In effect, you will have to find ways of letting your real self show without relying on your face to do the donkey-work in making friends.

Your previous personality does not determine your chances of changing faces, but figuring out new ways of communication will force some hitherto hidden aspects of your character more to the fore. Whereas before you may have relied on your looks in social situations, now your other attributes and qualities assume greater initial impact and have to be highlighted.

So try to take your new face as a positive force for bringing out the best in you and as a challenge for you and others to come to terms with.

Take Control of Your Future

I sometimes think that all facially disfigured people should receive Assertiveness Training as part and parcel of their rehabilitation along with other forms of treatment. Unfortunately, facial injuries often so complicate a person's life that there is little time or energy available to learn new ploys. Instead the pressing demands of home life, earning a living, financial security and other problems impose themselves, and the disfigured person leaves the hospital treatment regime very inadequately prepared for what he is destined to face outside.

Assertiveness is called for in so many areas: you have to discover how to hack through the undergrowth of medical jargon and not be satisfied with less than intelligible answers to your questions. You have to gain the respect of your surgeon, so that together you can plot out your future treatment. In all meetings with friends or strangers you have to let people know that you have sanity and worth. And in any future career you have to make your own way – your disfigurement is unlikely to help your chances.

Deciding on the surgical possibilities for your face is a key area where you have to take control: you (and those close to you) must try to establish a rapport with your surgeon and his team. In doing so, your future treatment can be worked out for your maximum benefit. Self-esteem can be much enhanced by facial improvements, but, as you may spend weeks recovering from the necessary operations, you have to be sure that you can influence how far and for how long the surgical interventions continue. There comes a point where you think you will not gain any more by further, time-consuming cosmetic work. Where that point is will be different in each case, but there is nothing to be gained by going on beyond it. When you can discuss this and, if necessary, persuade your surgeon accordingly, you have taken control. To do this you need a certain command of the relevant medical vocabulary, because without it you may find effective communication difficult. You may have some work to do to discover what the surgical opportunities are, so that you can put yourself in a position to contribute and even alter the course of your facial treatment.

Taking control is not confined to the hospital setting; that arena will come to play an increasingly small part in your life. The principle is of much wider relevance. As you start to circulate in public places again, you will come across many situations where there is unease among others as to how to behave in your presence. Again and again, you will have the opportunity to take control: it may be only a smile or offering to shake hands, but through that small gesture you have taken the initiative and asserted your acceptability.

So try to develop an assertive attitude of mind where you attempt to take control – maybe not full control – over your destiny. Although it sounds like a risky strategy, as the saying has it, 'Nothing ventured, nothing gained'.

Smarten Yourself Up

The damage to your face has transformed your view of yourself and the image you convey to others. You may not be very pleased about either of these developments. If you find yourself unattractive, what will others think of you? Unfortunately, miracle restorations are out of the question. You will be disfigured to some extent for the rest of your life. But you need not compound your disfigurement by letting other aspects of your outward appearance go into decline. In other words, it may even be a good move to uplift your valuation of yourself by ensuring that you present yourself as smart and organized in public.

Part of the problem all disfigured people confront is the feeling that their face is a mess, and, worse, that the mess can't quickly – or ever – be tidied up. Over some years it may be possible to put back some of the order and symmetry into your facial features through plastic surgery, with some scarring and discolouration remaining.

The mess that is your face should not spill over into the rest of your lifestyle. It should not become an excuse for shabbiness of dress or lack of attention to basic cleanliness. If either of these set in, you will fall from grace in the eyes of others, even if they might show a bit of understanding initially. More crucially, however, your own self-esteem is likely to drain away. If, on the other hand, you do take care to present a tidy appearance, you will strengthen your self-valuation. More importantly, perhaps, you will pleasantly surprise other people. This is particularly true for disfigured women: you may have lost what is considered your beauty, but you can still be attractive as stylish, neat, fashionable or just well-groomed.

The significance of feeling clean and tidy for morale hardly needs explanation. We all know that if we are feeling down and gloomy, a wash and brush-up will often bring on a brighter countenance. Equally, if we let our appearance go for a few days (perhaps when travelling), it does eventually take its toll on our mood. I can vouch for the validity of this principle even when you are in the very early hours after a serious accident or fire. The simple remedy of a hair wash skilfully administered to a prostrate patient does wonders for morale.

I am not suggesting that you should go out and spend a fortune on a new wardrobe. But you can achieve great psychological uplift by dressing well, by using make-up cleverly or by simply being clean and tidy. Although no great expense is called for, you may need to pay rather more attention to detail than before, perhaps. (Some who know me will find it laughable that I am advocating smartness, because my own rehabilitation took place in the years of long hair, beads and permissiveness in dress and much else. It might not have appeared to them that I was trying to be smart, but I was actually following the fashions of the day!)

A cautionary note is needed here: there is no possibility that clothes and cosmetics alone will enable you to change faces successfully. In some ways they are disguises that just put off the day when you take on your new face with confidence. They should not therefore be treated as more than minor aids. Cosmetics can be very effective in covering birthmarks, but they are rarely able to do more than tone down the blotchiness and extreme redness of the skin grafting or burns. They cannot recover the lost skin texture and will therefore be a poor disguise, however deftly applied. Cosmeticians do have a role in the recovery of damaged faces, however, and for some disfigured people make-up may be a fairly high priority, especially in the early days.

So don't let your tarnished face be reflected in shabby clothes and appearance. Put on a bright exterior and thereby boost your own confidence and other people's acceptance of you.

All these strategies sound so easy on paper, but in reality they may often conflict with your natural instincts. What I have sought to suggest is that your attitude to your disfigured face has to be, as far as possible, a positive one. Many set-backs and misfortunes may accompany your disfiguring accident. You may lose friends and the support of your family; you may receive a hostile public reception; you may lose your job and your career prospects; you may feel aggrieved and resentful at your plight and harbour grudges against those whom you hold responsible. Such disastrous personal views and experiences for someone trying to come to terms with a changed face would hardly seem to prompt a positive outlook. Yet it is surprising how a small word here or a bit of encouragement there, a new way of looking at the future or a more philosophical assessment of the past, can lead to adopting the type of positive approach that will enable you to change with your face.

There is no perfect answer or advice that will work for every disfigured person, but there are guide-lines. In addition to the strategies discussed above, there is another option; however, I believe it is one best avoided.

'Put a brave face on it'. This would involve trying courageously to tolerate your new face, accept its limitations, admit your reduced prospects, and fit into the slot reserved for the socially handicapped. There is no question that a certain amount of courage is called for in the process of changing faces. There are painful moments when a brave face is as much as you can possibly summon up. But to extend that response to your general behaviour and attitudes will not be enough to help you through.

During my hospitalization I can recall many visitors and letters from friends encouraging me to 'keep smiling'. Difficult advice when your face is highly swollen, but the message was to adopt a smiling attitude to my plight. None of them could predict how I was going to face up to my face – nor could I. Smiling was as hopeful as they could be. I think the advice gradually faded from use as I started to develop my own more positive strategies with their help.

This brings me to the last point. No strategy is ever devised in your head only. You have to talk to others; you have to seek help even if this involves dropping a lot of pride. Changing faces is not a process that you can go through on your own. You need constant reinforcement and encouragement.

To sum up, then: in taking the road from realizing your disfigurement towards a new full life, you will need:

– to constantly persuade yourself that you are not a write-off;
– to be realistic about your future;
– to see your disfigurement as a challenge to be overcome;
– to take control of many aspects of your life;
– to smarten yourself up;

but **not** be content just to put on a brave face.

CHAPTER 9

Getting Help from the Professionals

There was a week during my early patching-up treatment when, in order to aid eyelid grafting, my surgeon stitched my eyelids together. My arms and legs were strapped up, and I was completely helpless. Everything had to be done for me. It was a strange, eerie feeling. Only a few weeks before I had been completely self-motivated, self-reliant and self-sufficient. Now I had no choice but to accept that I needed help, a lot of help – it wasn't easy. I wanted to reject, yet I knew I shouldn't.

Becoming facially disfigured puts you at the receiving end of many people's love, care, encouragement, advice and sympathy, and your gratitude to them will be hard to express. Receiving this massive support places you suddenly in a new position, one that is at once uncalled for and yet one that you are obliged to accept. You will have to cultivate the art of receiving help, and of asking for it too.

Changing faces is a journey during which you gradually reduce your reliance on help and guidance, and re-establish your self-confidence and self-containment. Along the road you will receive some 'help' that you do not need, and you will seek other 'help' that will not be forthcoming. The art of helping is highly refined today, with many professional caring groups and agencies that are trained and experienced in giving the right type of help. Carers and helpers have to cultivate sensitive eyes and ears to know when their help is needed and when to give appropriate messages of encouragement. Many helpers will give you unexpected assistance.

You would be forgiven, for example, for thinking that physiotherapists would not have much to offer the facially disfigured –

no physical exercise needed, surely. Physiotherapists may be primarily concerned with physical therapy, but their role goes further. In helping to rebuild your lost muscles as a bed-bound facially injured person, they have to learn about your potentials and limits – how far to push, how best to cajole, how much to expect. Once they discover these capacities, they are then in a position to mobilize you.

Helping should always be for a purpose, but the art of helping is in learning when to listen and sympathize, and when to badger and persuade – 'a time to sit and a time to get you going'. And to be helped also demands that you treat the gift of assistance as a privilege to be respected and to serve a purpose.

The worst sort of helping comes over as an unconvincing, half-baked attempt based on a feeling that poor unfortunate people like the facially disfigured ought to receive a little to lessen their burden. And the worst sort of receiving takes all the care for granted, abuses it and wastes the energy that the helpers have devoted.

As a facially injured person, you will need many different forms of help at different stages in your recovery. The help may be asked for or it may be given freely and unconditionally, but its aim should be to liberate you from its receipt. If it encourages you to become dependent on some crutch or support, it will be less than ideal. Coming to terms with your disfigurement is a personal challenge to restore your independence and your self-esteem. In winning the battle, you will hopefully liberate others and help them to realize that the disfigured and disabled are real, interesting and self-motivated people who just happen to have damaged faces or are paralysed in part of their body.

There are many people and groups who may be able to offer you assistance after facial injury; some will do so in big ways, others in seemingly trivial ways. Some will feel they have tried hard to help and have achieved little; others will just fail to hit it off with you; and still others will want to help but be unable to find a suitable way of doing so.

This chapter surveys the various sources of help that may be relevant to you without making any judgements about which will be best in your situation. But before focusing on you and your needs, it is important that you do not ignore the fact that those around you, especially your family, may need just as much help, perhaps more, than you do in the aftermath of your disfigurement.

The various types of help could be grouped according to the time in your recovery when they might be most effectively given. There is, however, so much overlap between the groups that I have chosen to discuss them under three broad headings: physical, psychological and social/financial/legal.

Physical Help

Cosmetic creams and make-up. Facial disfigurement is a physical experience, and today's surgical skills are capable of reconstructing and rejuvenating your facial looks – but never perfectly. There will always be a degree of oddness in your appearance. How far you go with renovative surgery is a matter for debate between you and your surgeon, but beyond that, you may be able to make further significant improvements by using cosmetic creams and make-up. Disfigured men and women can gain greatly in confidence by wearing such camouflage, and, odd though it may feel (if you are a man!) its cosmetic effects can be impressive, especially in the early days after skin replacement, when your face will tend to be a mass of different coloured and textured skin.

In Britain, the Red Cross and other charities have established 'camouflage clinics' in some hospitals specializing in the treatment of the facially injured, and you can obtain advice and cosmetic prescriptions from the NHS. Most plastic surgery departments will be able to suggest contacts outside the hospital and may, if necessary, arrange for trained cosmeticians to come in and instruct you in the use of creams. Their application does need practice, and it is important that you persevere until you get the right blends and colour matches.

The great benefit of make-up is the toning-down effect it has on very conspicuous red scars. In fact, creams can also promote the desirable softening of the scar tissue prior to major plastic surgery and may also reduce the itchiness of hypertrophic scarring.

My own limited use of make-up came as a result of a chance remark by my surgeon, but I always felt it was like wearing a crusty, odd-looking mask that made my face very conspicuous. Instead, I favoured dark glasses, large-rimmed hats and scarves as camouflage, but they weren't exactly designer garments and were more attention drawing than attention deflecting. However, I was very attached to them for some years and felt very exposed if for some reason I was without them.

If you do concentrate on getting cosmetic help, you should not do so at the expense of other physical rehabilitation. Facial disfigurement is not in itself physically handicapping, and there is therefore no reason why you should not present a fit and/or elegant figure to the world. Indeed, if you do not, your facial oddness will be publicly seen as a symptom of your generally poor physical appearance. One major stepping-stone on my own journey to changing faces was to get back to playing squash, where I could assert my physical normality (sometimes much to my opponent's amazement).

Physiotherapy is an integral part of facial recovery, because by improving your physical strength and stamina you will experience a general 'well' feeling that will buoy you up and help you to make progress with your facial rehabilitation. Although physiotherapy plays only a small part in your physical restoration, in hospital it can often set the tone by persuading you that you have not completely lost all mobility, agility and dexterity. The aim of physiotherapy is not just to redevelop depleted muscles; it also aims to resuscitate demoralized minds and spirits by rejuvenating the patient's sense of his physical well-being.

Occupational therapy may be relevant to facial recovery because it aims to rekindle your physical co-ordination and your ability to concentrate on a task. The hours of doing nothing, especially in the early days of hospitalization, will take their toll. You may be virtually incapable of reading more than a page at a time or concentrating long enough to play a simple card-game. You may even find that you lose a certain amount of knowledge for lack of practice.

The tasks that occupational therapists will set up for you must be so designed as to reawaken your interest in using your brain and hands. They will challenge you to do seemingly impossible things, and they should persist, because your stamina will be very slight at first. By discussing your previous interests not only with you but also with your family, they should be able to contrive suitable stimuli. And when you do respond to them, you will start to take pride in achievement again, something that may have been missing.

Occupational therapists may be far more important in the journey from facial disfigurement than they – or you – may realize. Your future life and work are certainly very unlikely to rely on your physical attributes, damaged as they are. You may well need to make the most of your mental faculties, more than you would perhaps have done before your disfigurement. Indeed, part of an occupational therapist's role should be to help redirect your ideas about what you will and will not be able to do in the outside world, in conjunction with other professionals like social workers.

Both physiotherapy and occupational therapy tend to be of most value in the early recovery stage after facial injury, although even later on you may find that by asserting your physical abilities and skills, you will persuade others of your essential likeableness. The very moving BBC documentary about the Brazilian boy David Lopez/Jackson made just this point: despite his massive deformities, David's great sporting prowess won him respect and friends among his peers – 'Everyone wanted him in their team'. This is not just true in facial disfigurement: the feats of one-legged skiers, wheelchair athletes and one-armed golfers give the lie to their incompetence or physical limitations.

All of these examples point to the importance of raising your physical co-ordination and strength to new heights. Not everyone has to run a marathon or be a world-class rugger-player, though. Your own achievements may seem insignificant in this light, but that is irrelevant. The fact is that few people will expect someone looking like you to be able to *do* anything. Enjoy challenging them to see their own assumptions as absurd. By getting physical help, you can also shatter your own instincts that say the same sort of thing.

Psychological Help

Clinical Psychologists. There is a common confusion in the understanding of the word 'psychology'. It is the study of normal mental and emotional behaviour, in contrast to 'psychiatry', which focuses on mental diseases like schizophrenia or psychosis. Many psychological problems may arise from facial injuries, especially ones concerned with a disfigured person's self-identity.

Clinical psychologists are trained to assess and identify any problems associated with normal behaviour. So, for example, they might deal with the psychological consequences of being in a major fire: nightmares, guilt, depression. They may bring a variety of treatments to bear on these entirely natural problems, psychoanalysis and psychotherapy being two methods commonly used. But psychologists are not medically trained; they cannot prescribe drugs; and they do not claim to be able to treat psychiatric disorders of the mind on their own.

In the process of changing faces, you and your family will confront a whole series of new experiences, new challenges and new problems. Trying to reconcile yourself to what has happened to you, trying to prepare yourself for taking your disfigurement into public places, trying to work out with your family whether life will ever be tolerable or enjoyable again, trying to shake off the demoralization you feel about your future – these and many other trials await you along the road to facial rehabilitation.

The aim of clinical psychologists is to get you to recognize and admit to having a problem, to trace it back to its roots and then to create a treatment regime that will help you to resolve it. They are not the only psychological experts that you may come into contact with: social workers, religious pastors, marriage guidance counsellors and others may all have psychological skills, even if they don't have the big initials after their names. You don't have to make use of their help; you may not do so consciously anyway. Their art is in bringing your anxieties, fears and frustrations to the surface without deliberately forcing the issue. Once you have started to talk, you are probably halfway towards finding solutions to problems that you may not have even realized were troubling you.

Many people can provide psychological help if you trust them with your confidences, but you are the one in control. The skill of the psychologist is in leading you up to the point when you do let go and unburden. 'Counselling' often amounts to the counselled healing themselves. In this sense your friends and family may be able to offer you assistance, but they may lack the crucial emotional distance from you that is needed for really sound advice to be given and received willingly.

Nowadays clinical psychologists are often attached to burns units (and other hospital departments caring for the facially injured), and this enables them to make contact with you early on. Just as importantly, they can establish a link with your family, offer themselves as willing and sensitive healers of emotional wounds and start the process of rebuilding your shattered life. This is their professional job, and, while other staff on the burns unit may also hear your ups and downs and gain your confidence, the psychologist has the special role of getting you to face up to your situation.

Some of their questions can be really tough. 'How do you think X feels about your face?' 'Why do you feel ashamed?' These may be questions to which as yet you do not have any answers, and, even if you did, you would prefer to keep them to yourself. Having said that, the psychological release you may feel by just speaking around the subjects can be immense – it's a relief to find someone you can talk to about them.

The taboo of facial disfigurement was for so long so strong that discussing it was ruled out for many disfigured people. They were expected to put on a brave face and be outwardly cheerful through it all. The advent of modern psychological methods changed that. Now, if anything, you are expected to be openly soul-searching, and that too may prove difficult for people not used to offloading their deeper feelings to others.

Social workers. If clinical psychologists can give you the chance to come to terms with your new situation while in hospital, you may be left somewhat bereft of help once outside. Social workers, who often dovetail the resources of the hospital and the local community, are your most likely source of psychological aid in your life beyond the hospital. If they have made the effort to contact you and your family, they may be able to predict and therefore prevent some of the worst effects of re-entering the social world. They may be able to forestall marriage problems, for example, by referring you to a marriage guidance counsellor, and they may be able to reduce some of the considerable strain on your family by helping everyone to work effectively together.

Many burns units have made a major effort in recent years to offer an 'out-reach' service for their ex-patients, the aim being to provide a continuity of care and a source of succour and support. Psychologist, social worker plus, perhaps, a senior nurse and even a plastic surgeon make themselves available to the recently discharged disfigured person. There may well be certain areas of your rehabilitation that are not going well – your relations with the opposite sex, for example. To have regular contact with a specialist may give you a confidence that would otherwise have been missing.

Self-help groups. Some facially disfigured people find that they can benefit enormously from sharing their experiences in self-help groups of people with similar problems. There are a number of such groups in Britain (see the section on Useful Organizations), but many hospitals aim to run such groups as part of their standard rehabilitation treatment. Ex-patients are encouraged to come back to discuss how they are faring, to share their triumphs and chew over their disasters.

The great merit of these groups is the common realization that facial disfigurement has befallen others, that you are not alone and that others have struggled with similar problems. As long as the sessions are well directed by a skilled counsellor, the risk of overdoing the unpleasant social experiences can be minimized and a positive approach adopted. There is also a lot to be gained by non-counsellor-directed discussions in and out of hospitals. Fellow patients or disfigured people can give you a tremendous psychological uplift, as long as they are not riddled with bitterness about their position.

It has always seemed to me rather disappointing that the most famous self-help group of all for the facially burned, the Guinea Pig Club for burned airmen of the Second World War, has not spread its wings and enlarged its membership and its impact. It still meets for an annual reunion, although it is now largely composed of people of retirement age. In its heyday after the last war, the Guinea Pigs had a high profile and, a very strong camaraderie; as a club, they behaved as if all members were facially normal. The stiff upper lip attitude was the spirit of the age, and they probably didn't openly discuss personal or psychological problems.

One of the most notable self-help groups for the facially disfigured in Britain today is the 'Let's Face It' group, formed by Christine Piff after her recovery from facial cancer and her rehabilitation with a prosthesis. The encouragement and mutual support that such groups can bring is undeniable, and they can usefully complement the work of social workers, other professionals and your family.

The first few months after hospital discharge are likely to be the hardest. Your feeling of isolation may be strongest, and your resolution to adopt some of the strategies suggested in this book may need constant reinforcement. Your family may be able to give a tremendous amount, but neither they nor the caring professions may, in your view, really know what it's like to be facially disfigured. That is where the support group of fellow sufferers can come into its own.

Social/legal/financial help

Becoming facially disfigured poses a number of practical problems. If these are not cleared up, doubts and suspicions may linger and adversely affect your recovery. If you were involved in a major disaster, the large number of people affected will ensure that considerable public interest is aroused in what arrangements are made for you and your family's future. This may not be so in the case of smaller incidents, and it is therefore important that you seek out authoritative help.

The common problems are many. What are the financial consequences for you and your family of your disfigurement? Can anything be done immediately to help to ease the financial burden? What about compensation? Who was legally liable for what happened to you? What are your employment prospects after such a facially disfiguring injury? Will your employer or school welcome you back?

Most of these are definitely issues that initially fall into the domain of your social worker, who should be able to ascertain fairly swiftly what social security benefits or assistance you could receive. The social worker may also get in touch with your employer where appropriate and establish your employment outlook. He should also be able to smooth out any anxieties you may have about the care of your family during your hospitalization.

Many loose ends will need to be tied up, and you may need to find someone to do the tying. Delegating may seem strange, but it is essential. If you are not satisfied with your social worker, it may be worth approaching a specialist. For financial advice, for example, consider contacting an accountant, who may have greater expertise in the relevant area.

On legal matters it is wise to go immediately and directly to a solicitor, and entrust him with all the difficulties that may arise in the minefield of the law. The possibilities for obtaining some sort of compensation are far greater in Britain today than ever before, and certainly enormous insurance premiums are paid by employers and firms of all sorts in anticipation of claims for damages. Legal fees incurred are often recoverable. Your solicitor will also be able to take any pressure off you and your family from the media or the police, and can therefore allow you all to come to terms privately with the effects of your facial injuries.

The issue of your future work or occupation will be left very much on your shoulders, and advice on what would be the best direction for you may be hard to come by. Clearly there may be some jobs and careers that will be ruled out after your disfigurement, but your knowledge of what is on offer may be limited. You may be well advised to take some kind of retraining or obtain some extra qualifications in order to stand a better chance of getting employment. In the first instance it is probably worth asking your social worker to put you in contact with a suitable careers adviser.

Ultimately changing faces is your challenge, but by sharing your anxieties and practical problems you can benefit from the advice and experience of people who have helped others on their journeys and may be able to help you too. You may be able to get help from many sources on the road to facial recovery. Don't expect miracles – the helpers are only human. However, if you've got a problem, there are people who can help you, so don't suffer in silence.

CHAPTER 10

Are People Scared of You?

Every facially disfigured person has to get used to a set of very common reactions in people they meet: Staring, Curiosity, Anguish, Recoil, Embarrassment and Dread – the SCARED syndrome. In a way, SCARED sums up the feelings of people meeting you and your face. They are literally scared of the unknown: how can they possibly communicate with you? They've never met anyone like you before, and they are scared of having to talk to you, scared of hurting you, scared of asking questions, scared of looking at you . . .

One secret of changing faces is to realize that *you* have to help them to break out of their 'scared-ness' and meet you face to face. I will try to explain how you can do this by considering each aspect of being scared. Each element runs over into another: recoil (when people shy away from you) will often be close to embarrassment, for example. You will find that many people you meet will suffer from a mixture of several ingredients, often all of them.

Staring

You will be able to sense that your face, and hands too perhaps, are being scrutinized; you will develop a sixth sense that tells you when you are being examined. If you look at the starer, he is likely either to turn away in confusion or to try to get into conversation about something else – to change the subject. By looking at him, you will confuse or embarrass him, which may make future contact more difficult. So you have to get used to being inspected and you have to put up with being stared at, because it is essential that people become accustomed to your new face. People you meet need to have the chance to take a good look at you.

Friends of mine have sometimes commented that they have felt protective towards me when people are staring, because it often seems so obvious and thoughtless. There are different sorts of staring – some can be quite malicious – but, for the most part, your face is an object of interest and information. I try never to make anyone feel bad about staring at me – well, almost never – but there are times when you can't help feeling irritated by persistent, blatant staring, and you may have to register your annoyance. But most staring is simply information-gathering.

Many disfigured people turn away from being stared at, a natural reaction, although it is one that can suggest you have something rather unpleasant to hide. Staring is a necessary preparation for many 'normals' before they can look you in the face, let alone the eye. For this reason, if you are in a social gathering, many people will stare prior to talking to you. From across the room, the starer hopes he is not being noticed, but your sixth sense will keep you informed.

I play squash to a fairly high standard in a local club, and I am frequently aware of eyes inspecting me from the balcony. Here I am, active and doing something 'normal'. Obviously in the middle of a game I can't react directly to the staring, but just by being seen to do an ordinary activity, I am conveying a message. Occasionally I find my opponents rather overawed by my normality. 'Surely people who look like you can't play squash?' I can hear them saying to themselves.

There are various ploys that can be quite effective at deterring staring if you are that unhappy with it. You can make direct but unmalicious eye-to-eye contact, indicating that you are quite capable of looking straight at them and have nothing to hide. Or again, staring can be met by joining conversation – pick a subject on which you think the onlookers will have some strong opinions and be interested in their answers. Before you know it, they will have forgotten their staring and be immersed in telling their stories. You will have to keep up the conversation until you judge it right to help them ask the big question: 'What happened to you?'

Staring can simply be accepted as part of the disfigurement

package: changing faces is partly to do with getting used to being an object of scrutiny wherever you go. In the early days of re-entry into your world, you will find people's inspection of your facial damage very invasive. Their eyes will feel like drills, adding psychological pain to your physical injuries. Even twenty years on, I do turn away from staring sometimes because of its intensity. This is particularly true with children, who can become uninhibitedly transfixed in their staring (see Chapter 11).

Judging when to turn away, when to allow the staring to continue or when to stare back is not easy. It largely depends on whether you are disconcerted by it. There is no way that you can avoid public scrutiny, and my advice is to take as much as you can without overreacting to it. Now I am almost oblivious of it for much of the time except in very crowded areas, like London Underground trains. The most frustrating thing about being stared at is that in only a few instances do you get the chance to explain that you are quite a normal person underneath. But you can devise ways of conveying your personality without relying on your facial looks.

Curiosity

'I hope you don't mind me asking, but what happened to you?' Point-blank questions such as this are surprisingly common and are often accompanied by an explanation like, 'I knew someone who was terribly badly burned in the war.' Curiosity often can't be bottled up, and the fact they knew someone who looked like you provokes very direct questioning.

While it can be quite a welcome change to be questioned uninhibitedly and talk straightforwardly about your injuries, sometimes it can be too much. In a public place everyone's ears suddenly prick up as they strain to hear your answers, and the room goes quiet. There is little option: you have to respond as favourably as you can to this inquisition. You may not feel like giving much away, in which case you must have a shorthand version of your story that you can fluently produce. Unfortunately, curious people are rarely satisfied by this and will probe with more: 'When is your next plastic surgery going to be done?' If you are reluctant to give anything away, you can always brush people off with a curt 'none of your business', but I would suggest that their curiosity is actually a good opportunity for you to spread the word about your 'normality' and thereby encourage them to look at other disfigured (or disabled) people in a more favourable light. This means being unusually frank with them – 'unusually' in the sense that before your disfigurement you wouldn't have dreamed of telling your personal story to strangers or very new acquaintances. Usually you would expect to observe social conventions of 'getting to know you' before any personal details are exchanged. Changing faces means living in an unusual way for the rest of your life.

Responding to curiosity gives you an opening: you can illustrate by your replies that your disfigured appearance is no guide to your inner character. Friends of mine are quite shocked, I think, when they hear me chatting away to complete strangers about myself. But if I am not open, I stand less chance of being taken seriously, and in general, I have found that openness helps to lay foundations for friendships.

My disfigurement is so very obvious that curiosity is inevitable. It is ironic that often the people who are the most curious have many problems of their own, though less conspicuous ones. They often wish someone would ask them leading questions, so they can offload their problems. Their curiosity about my disfigurement turns out to be their cry for help.

Anguish

Some people you meet will feel, and may even show, profound anguish about your loss of facial good looks and the suffering they imagine you have been through. They feel your pain intensely, sometimes to the extent of breaking down in your presence. Their deep sense of sympathy for you, and with you, is really very touching, but they may feel so overwhelmed by it that their attitude and behaviour towards you can become inhibited.

Instead of expressing their anguish, they may freeze up in your presence (and be very unhappy about doing so). Alternatively, their sympathy can be demonstrated in fulsome shows of pity lavished on you at every turn. In both these extremes you have to help them to express themselves and work the sympathy out.

In the first case, where their anguish makes them freeze up, you must understand their difficulty: they don't want you to see how sad they are for you, for fear that you will feel even worse. But you can see it in their eyes. They are mourning for you, for what you've lost, but they are afraid to cry or say how sorry they are. The temptation in such circumstances is to state the simple 'I'm OK' line and hope that this reassurance will be sufficient to let their anguish subside to tolerable, less immediate levels and allow them to act normally towards you. Sometimes this works, occasionally with a passing remark from them like, 'Oh, you are so brave'. When they come to terms with you and converse without inhibition, your 'I'm OK' statement may need some elaboration. Unfortunately, the anguished tend to take the 'I'm OK' reassurance as just a valiant effort on your part to put a brave face on it, and they just don't believe that you can ever possibly be OK again. If anything, their anguish deepens. What they need is to be able to believe by your actions that you don't feel bitter or resentful of your lot. If you can genuinely show this, their anguish will be dissipated, because they will realize that you don't want or need sympathy.

Bitterness is not easy to quell in yourself (as was discussed in Chapter 3 on coping with the causes of your disfigurement), so to transmit your lack of it to others is particularly difficult. Probably the best way to convince others is to be full of life, interested in what is happening, in the latest gossip and news, and to able to crack jokes at your own expense. Laughter is a good way to break down deeply felt sympathy without abusing it. It conveys the fact that life can still be, and often is, fun. What, even if you're facially disfigured? Yes. And once you have broken the ice with a face-splitting joke or comment or amusing reminiscence, you can be serious if they want to be. In other words, you are lightening the darkness of their anguish and helping them to help you by being more than just speechless and sad.

At the other extreme, you may occasionally meet overpowering displays of anguish when someone almost swamps you with messages of sympathy, maybe flowers or other gifts, and treats you as one of life's unfortunates. I have felt positively embarrassed by this sort of extravagant pity – and also irritated. But it is important to understand the genuine concern behind the heavy-handedness. Your disfigured face may be a trigger for some people to show their caring side, but they do so rather over-elaborately. What you have to do is tone it down. All this can be rather tricky. The more you try to demonstrate how well you have recovered, and thus contest your assumed need for sympathy, the more you seem to be rejecting the sympathy. In its overdone form, sympathy firmly burdens you with the status of 'handicapped for life', which is certainly not what you want. You must try to turn the sympathy to constructive uses.

One way of doing this is to lift the sorrowful atmosphere by asking for positive ideas for the future. Well-directed sympathy is not mollycoddling; it is a listening, helpful support when you need it. It does not force itself on you, yet you can draw on its warmth in your downhearted moods. So the oversympathetic person has to be asked to be a positive aid rather than a patting and pitying weight on you. Once they realize they can really help by seeing the results, their value to you increases considerably.

Anguish is not easy to allay, but if you do not try to do so, facial disfigurement can seem a very depressing and saddening experience. You can start to wallow in your misfortune. This is why, right from the start, people who meet you need to adopt an understanding role as listeners and also a positive approach to your future. Strangely enough, sometimes you can help them to do so.

Recoil

Facial oddness is a shock to the beholder. Recoil is a very natural reaction to it. There will always be people who blink hard at the sight of you, take a step backwards, avert their eyes, gasp, refuse to sit next to you, shield their children from you and by many other actions register their backing off. None of these responses should surprise you. You have to learn to take them in your stride; like staring, they are part of the disfigured's lot. And like staring, they should not go unnoticed or without some reaction from you.

This is not a call for heroics or wild extroversion. You cannot do much to lessen the shock for people. Your face is abnormal, and it will take people's breath away. But what you may be able to do is to make those who recoil come back by indicating that you are another normal human being underneath, able to smile, laugh and speak. This is much easier to do if you are in the company of normal-faced friends, because they, by their acceptance of you, will signal your sanity to others. When you are on your own, it is a matter of finding sensitive and effective ways of reassurance. Eye contact is one way of restoring someone's belief in you, but this is difficult where the recoil is shown by a complete refusal to look you in the face. A direct approach is important, because it shows you have nothing to hide.

The following incident, recalled by an old friend whom I hadn't seen since my accident, illustrates this. 'The doorbell rang. I opened the door of my flat and on the darkened landing, I saw a tall, unrecognizable figure wearing a hat. My initial reaction was to recoil. I didn't recognize you but even in the dark I could see something wasn't right. It only lasted a split second, because you spoke immediately, stuck out your hand and my initial reaction of fear/horror? was gone. You stepped into the light and my first reaction was replaced with one of curiosity – finally I was seeing for myself what had been described to me by others who had seen you before I did.'

Another friend recalls the party where we first met. 'I had seen you in the room not knowing who you were and wondering how I could cope if we were introduced. However, we started talking about our children, and I found it quite difficult at first looking at you directly – but as time went on this worry disappeared and I realized how unimportant your appearance was.'

These two examples show how you can adopt quite an aggressive stance to your disfigurement by wearing it with an outward show of confidence. Being upset by other people's recoil might be your spontaneous reaction, but you need not be demoralized. Even if you do feel nervous at first, your confidence will grow as you successfully bring some people back from their recoil. You can, at least, give everyone something to think about.

Embarrassment

Perhaps the most common reaction to being with a disfigured person was summed up by a friend of mine: 'My overriding recollection is of being unrelaxed and ill at ease with you at first, because I was trying to pretend that I was looking at somebody who wasn't facially disfigured, rather as I might do to someone with a nasty spot on their nose.' Unrelaxed, ill at ease, awkward, confused – many people will experience this sort of reaction to you, for the simple and understandable reason that they don't quite know what is expected of them when meeting you. Just as you are very self-conscious of your face, the people you meet will also become very self-conscious of their own behaviour, language and attitude to you. Another friend commented, 'I'd have liked to be able to look closely but was too self-conscious to do so – and too concerned as to what was the right course: to stare could be embarrassing; to be seen to be almost avoiding looking could be worse. Perhaps I was thinking more about me than about you!'

The dilemma that you face in trying to dissolve this awkwardness is that it stems from other people's unfamiliarity with facial disfigurement and their basic lack of knowledge about its causes and implications. People can feel quite shy on meeting you and be particularly worried at not knowing whether your speech or brain had also been impaired in your accident. As a disfigured person, your problem is how you can calm the anxiety of the people you meet without making them feel even more awkward.

If, for example, you offer them too much too quickly in the form of a full-scale account of your particular facial problems, they may be even more embarrassed, because they are anxious that it must be painful for you to explain it all. You have, therefore, to be sure that they are ready, and that you have conquered your own painful thoughts, because this is the key to resolving their uncertainty.

Your aim should be to help them ask the questions that are on the tip of their tongue and to volunteer answers with no scruples. Only occasionally will it be worth giving a complete explanation of your facial damage. You will probably be pleasantly surprised by how little information people need in order to gain confidence in talking and relating to you. Often all they want to know is that your facial injuries are under treatment, that some surgical options have been investigated and that behind the scars is an active mind and a normal set of emotions.

Your 'problem' is highly conspicuous. It is out in the open for all to see, in marked contrast to the psychological, emotional and internal scars and problems from which some people suffer. This can be to your advantage: other people see that something has happened to you, and you then have a golden opportunity to widen their understanding of it. Less conspicuous 'problems' are far more difficult to talk out and as a result may fester and deepen.

There is great value for all disfigured people in talking about their experiences in an open and honest way. Your disfigurement may be no easier to live with, but by talking with others, you can learn much about their fears and anxieties on meeting you. And this should enable you to build up a picture in your mind of how others see you, embarrassment and all. You can draw on this knowledge and shape your behaviour accordingly when you next meet embarrassment – and the same process is true for any other response.

However, I have assumed that this willingness to be open is something that comes easily. It doesn't to some disfigured people. They consider their recovery to be a painful private affair that they would rather forget and certainly not impose on anyone else. If this is the case with you, you will have to tackle embarrassment in some other way: perhaps you will have to back away from such awkward moments and limit your social contacts to those with whom you feel confident, a brother or sister, for example. But living with disfigurement in this withdrawn way will certainly confirm the assumptions that other people will automatically hold about you: that you lack the personality and courage to overcome the social ostracism that your facial disfigurement brings. Sadly, this route of self-imposed exile is sometimes chosen by the disfigured. But you need not sacrifice your future if you can bring yourself out and take some risks in what you do.

I sometimes have the impression that people are embarrassed to meet me because they are so surprised that someone with a face like mine is doing anything with his life. The assumption is that people with scarred faces don't show them in public – and it is highly embarrassing for everyone when they do. The logical inference of this is that disfigured people ought not to show their faces . . .

There is undoubtedly much public education needed to inform the public eye and mind, so that there is more understanding of disfigurement. In the early years after the Second World War, when the sight of burned fighter pilots and air-raid victims was relatively common, public awareness and knowledge of facial damage made it so much easier for the disfigured to be generally accepted. But however effective the educational effort may be, the fact remains that people will be confused by your appearance, and you must take positive steps to quell their embarrassment. And in the process of doing so, you will be amazed to find that you have done much to relieve your own embarrassment.

Dread

Your disfigurement will go before you. People will be warned that your face is badly scarred – and this warning is neither undesirable nor preventable. The problem is that it can completely dominate people's attitude and behaviour towards you. Their imagination is given free rein, and all kinds of unsightly facial images present themselves in their mind's eye, often complete with a personality stereotype to match. For them the prospect of meeting you may become quite dreadful; they go through mental contortions to try to conjure a way of avoiding meeting you face to face. It's not that they are worried about being embarrassed: it is a simple fear of the unknown and the ugly.

As the disfigured party, you can have little direct influence on this sort of terror, because you have not met the fearful person yet. You have therefore to depend on the good judgement of your friends, on your reputation or on taking immediate action to dispel the fears at your first meeting. The only other recourse is to rely on the gradual dawning of public understanding, which will be a slow and uncertain route.

Friends and social contacts are the conveyers of messages about you to total strangers or old friends who have yet to see you. What they tell of your facial looks and your outlook on your past and future will greatly influence how the rest of the world sees you – or expects to see you. If their portrait is of a melancholy person weighed down by the awful legacy of facial damage, they will give the impression that your face dominates and diminishes your life. They will have to report to others that your underlying personality is so shattered by your tarnished self-image that it is barely of significance. They presume that the horridness of your face clouds your inner self, and your external deformities are really all there is to report. The rest of you is non-existent. This is a disastrous thumbnail sketch to use in preparing a reaction to you. Is it surprising that the meeting is viewed with dread? You have triggered fear: your face has gone before you.

How much different this could – and can – be if you are able to inspire reports of interest, respect, even admiration. If people can say, 'She's coping wonderfully', however exaggerated this may be, it is certainly preferable to reports of 'It is awful to look at.' The point is that in any preparatory warnings your character should be reported as overcoming your facial disadvantages.

I do not mean to suggest that you can completely eliminate people's fear of meeting you. As you will remember, before you were disfigured you didn't find it easy to anticipate meeting a handicapped person or someone who had suffered a stroke, for example. You may have been nervous of saying or doing the wrong thing, or of being rather repulsed by their physical difficulties. Dread is such a common anticipatory feeling that all facially disfigured people should prepare themselves to cope with it in others, but not in a passive set-piece way. You cannot hide your face, but you can indicate that its oddities are not as dreadful as they look.

Throughout the first few minutes of conversation with someone who has been dreading meeting you, you will realize that they are only half listening; the rest of their attention is devoted to looking you over minutely. And then they will abruptly announce, 'It's nothing like as bad as I thought it would be' – 'it' being your face. This could prompt a brief explanation from you of what 'it' feels like or is destined to look like after surgery. And then the conversation can return to 'normal'. They have been put at ease. What was all the fuss about? The next time such a meeting is in the offing, far less dread will be experienced, making it easier all round.

CHAPTER 11

Children Reacting

In the previous chapter, I suggested that facial disfigurement often prompts a response from within the SCARED range (Staring, Curiosity, Anguish, Recoil and Dread). Indeed, the reactions that fall within this range are so common that you will become better and better prepared and gradually work out effective counters to each component of the syndrome. At first some of the ploys might seem like risky, untried manoeuvres, but with practice they will become almost automatic, and you will find it easier to pick the right tactic to suit each situation. There are some groups of people, though, whose responses are likely to cause you considerable difficulty and embarrassment. However well you have adapted to disfigurement and however experienced you are at coping with people's reactions, meetings with children can often make you feel uncomfortable.

Facial oddness is particularly fascinating to children. Hardly any child between the ages of two and ten years will have much prior understanding or knowledge about scarred, marked or deformed faces. Even faces with beards are viewed as abnormal by those children who happen not to have met many bearded men in their circle of family friends. So when you meet children, the way they react to your odd face is completely unpredictable. This means that you have to be ready for almost anything. If the child has been prepared for the shock of seeing your face – and many parents will have chosen to warn them – this can sometimes make their instant reaction less impulsive, athough it rarely reduces the chance of you being caught out by their unexpected behaviour.

Frequently children will take you at face value. Your disfigured face is what they see and interpret, and they will act on this interpretation, which will, in all likelihood, be based on some very simple notions of good and bad. There is definitely an age, from say three to five years, when the correlation of good with handsomeness, and bad with ugliness, is very strong. These basic image associations are learned very early on and are not challenged until most children are beyond five years. The first childhood books and fairy-tales work on very clear moral principles.

Your disfigured face may therefore provoke fear if looked at by any in this age group, the sort of fear that sends a child running screaming to find mummy! This can be exceedingly embarrassing, especially if it happens in a public place, because the screams will immediately draw the attention of other people to you. You will wish you could curl up or vanish at such a terrible experience. It can transform a pleasant event, like a wedding reception, into a miserable occasion for you.

Your discomfort will be due to your feeling of shame at having scared a child. You can take comfort, if you like, in the knowledge that you will not be the only frightening thing the child has seen – even jovial Father Christmas frequently gets this terror-stricken reaction from small children. There is very little you can do about it, except seek to reassure 'mummy' that *you* are only superficially wounded. You will certainly find it well nigh impossible to reassure the child – and the more you try, the more he may howl. So standing away is your best strategy.

Fear is one extreme of the unpredictable reactions in children. At the other end of the spectrum is their supreme openness. You will come across some children who will ask you the most point-blank, uninhibited questions, often in highly public places. The straightforward question, 'What's wrong with your face?' will shatter the most tranquil of situations. At such moments the parent or other person in charge will zoom in instantly to try to remove the child. As adults, they may be too embarrassed by the whole scene to feel able to listen to your answer, and they will prefer to whisk the child away before you have a chance to respond. However understandable this parental instinct, it is unfortunate, because it deprives the child (and the parent too!) of gaining appreciation that not everyone looks the same, and that people should not be judged on the basis of their looks.

Furthermore the parent is actually creating or reinforcing the false impression in the child's mind that disfigured people are suspicious and should be avoided.

If, on the other hand, parents are prepared to listen to your answer, they give you the opportunity to give a clear, child-level account of why you look as you do. You will not need a lengthy explanation: a few well-chosen words will count for a lot. You have to draw on and direct the child's basic knowledge: 'I was in a fire . . . then hospital . . . Have you ever been to hospital?' You will be amazed by how much and how quickly children appreciate your plight. Even comparatively young children are quite capable of understanding some of the technical details like skin grafts – and quite incapable of knowing when to stop their inquisition! Children are full of questions. You have to be prepared to answer them, or even to offer the answers to unasked questions.

In between fear and open questioning are a number of other uninhibited reactions to your face. Staring quite fixedly and unconsciously is one. But less acceptable is the occasional incident when older children in gangs behave quite objectionably by daringly calling you names that they have either invented or heard elsewhere. Such behaviour is horribly abusive, and your choice of how to respond is a no-win one: either you passively submit to the name-calling or get irritable and display your anger. Neither approach is likely to feel very satisfactory. This kind of abuse is rarely hostile in a malicious sense, but unsupervised youths in gangs seem to know when they have caught an adult in his weak spot and will play on it unmercifully. So you will be able to spot trouble coming if you see a group approaching or if you are walking in their direction; where possible, it might be wise to take avoiding action.

Thankfully, more usual than this offensive behaviour is when children are a bit wary of you. They are just nervous and unsure – quite understandable reactions that will show themselves in backing off. But the great thing with children is how quickly they can be won over once they see you as you really are rather than as you look. A few words of reassurance can sometimes settle a child, but it is better still to distract them. Most children are easily diverted. A new game, questions about themselves or their family

– any of these can often bridge the gap, and before long they will be playing with you and your face won't matter.

The question that often arises for parents of small children who are about to meet you for the first time is whether or not to prepare them for your odd-looking face. This is very much a matter of judging each child on the basis of his sensitivity and shyness. The problem is that if parents do not inform, the child may be shocked into fear or tears, thereby ruining the meeting. On the other hand, by warning the child in advance, unnecessary worry may be created in the child's mind, and he may not be able to act naturally when meeting you.

Often it is the parents who are nervous about what you will feel like if one of their children pays obvious attention to your looks or starts quizzing you. So their prior warnings are really as much attempts to prevent the awkwardness they will feel as they are shock-absorbers for their children. One parent remembers a most embarrassing episode – 'I was in the kitchen and you were with Tommy, aged four, in the sitting-room. He suddenly asked you all sorts of questions about what your face felt like and your hand with its missing fingers . . . I was dying inside. You encouraged him to come and feel your face and hand and had quite a conversation about it. From that time onwards I noticed he was no longer worried.'

There is no doubt that being disfigured does complicate your relations with children, even ones who grow up alongside you. A nephew of mine was born around the time of my accident. As I went through the course of plastic surgery, my face was actually changing, and his anxiety grew. When he was about four years old, he became very afraid of clowns, and it was a while before his parents realized that he thought their faces were actually grotesque in reality and not just masks and make-up. Sessions with face paints seemed to sort this out.

The most distressing times are when children refuse to sit at the same table as you or even come to your house. Just reading about these sorts of incident may depress you, but facing up to them is part of changing faces. Although your facial looks may not be tolerable to some children during a particular phase in their life, they will grow out of it. You must change too, so that you can live with these set-backs.

You will suffer sometimes; you will wonder whether it would be better to avoid children for good. But you can develop perfectly sound relationships with them if you are patient and open. Above all, make the most of the chance to broadcast to those children what is or isn't in a face; in so doing, you can help them to see early on that people's facial appearances are no indication of character and make a small contribution to improving the lot of disfigured people everywhere.

Now that I have children of my own, I am fascinated and sometimes embarrassed by the reactions of their friends to me and my face. Some don't appear to notice at all, while others are wary. One child said to her father after meeting me, 'Is he really their daddy? He doesn't look like them and they don't look like him.' Perhaps that is just as well!

CHAPTER 12

Being in a Crowd

Meeting and being in crowds is a curious experience if you are disfigured. You have conflicting feelings about whether the crowd is reassuring or hostile. On the one hand, your facial disfigurement may be hardly significant in a crowd, and you can actually enjoy an anonymity that you are not able to experience in face-to-face contacts. There may be a few eyes examining you, but you don't need to respond; you can simply move with the crowd and almost forget your problems.

Crowds can feel very threatening to many disfigured people, however. You may feel isolated and open to ridicule, and you fear that your facial oddness will cause people to categorize you as 'thick' or 'mentally retarded'. You will be anxious to refute such imputations, and yet in a busy crowd there is no way of doing so. As a result you avoid crowds, and any public gathering is a potential hazard for you.

This conflict in how you, as a disfigured person, approach crowds should become easier as time passes, because you will gain more confidence in wearing your new face and you will learn how to cope with other people's reactions to it. But certainly in the early days of disfigurement, you will feel you want to avoid crowds and may be reluctant to let yourself be judged by them.

The escapist urge will be reinforced if you are unfortunate enough to suffer any distasteful experiences in crowds. For example, a group of people in a crowd who are somewhat the worse for alcohol find Dutch courage and start goading and jeering at you. Standing up to this distasteful behaviour could have the adverse effect of geeing up the hostility even more, so the safest solution is for you to withdraw quickly and quietly. Once you have been through any such horror, you will dread being exposed in public places such as buses, trains or football crowds, and you may be too shaken to venture out for some time. If you are in a group of disfigured or disabled people, you may be even more open to the butt-end of some unpleasant remarks. Being in a crowd with normal-faced friends will almost certainly protect you from abuse and assure your integrity; the very fact of being with a normal-looking person will give you credibility.

Learning how to carry your disfigured face in a crowd is one important part of changing faces, and here you can gain immensely by having a companion who is not disfigured. I can remember going with a friend to a league football match at a large London stadium not long after my discharge from hospital. He acted as a kind of shield for me, probably without realizing it. In effect, I hid behind his normality and enjoyed the social acceptance that being with him brought to me. Other friends have played similar roles in many circumstances, although I did not ask them to do so, and it is unlikely that they appreciated the help they were giving me.

If you try to tackle crowds on your own at the outset, you are more likely to give yourself unnecessary heart-ache. Don't be down-hearted if you don't have a suitable companion, for it can be done. In such circumstances your aim should be to carry off your disfigurement with as much confidence as you can.

Initially you may feel happier covering yourself up with dark glasses, make-up, hats, scarves or other gear. These disguises perform the role of your non-existent companion: they shield you from the full blast of public attention. Or so you think. Actually they probably attract more attention, because your attire is so bizarre. Nevertheless, if they do serve the purpose of enabling you to step out in public places, they are justifiable. They are not long-term solutions, though.

Throwing off the trappings of your disguise will be a liberating moment, because it will signal to you, and to the crowd, that you can take the full force of public attention with no need for shields or filters. Once you have reached this stage, your ability to live in and almost enjoy crowds will increase immensely, and you may even start to thrive on your noticeability!

The most difficult crowds for the disfigured to venture into are those where appearance plays a significant role: discothèques, night-clubs, social functions, beaches and swimming-pools. Not only does your oddness stand out very starkly from the smart and hyper-attractive people around you, but you feel the implied slurs. 'Should someone looking like you really be allowed to lower the tone of these sorts of surroundings?' or 'You aren't pretty enough to be seen among us.' Nothing may be said, but the looks tell all.

There will be occasions when you sense a hesitancy on the part of a restaurant, for example, to allow you in. If the restaurateur is seen to be catering for non-beautiful people, he may worry that his restaurant's status could slip. Would he do the same if he knew you were Nikki Lauda, the racing driver, burned but a celebrity? Another reason given to prevent you entering or using a particular place is that your face will upset the other clients and customers.

My inclination is to make the most of social situations by being so obviously at home and enjoying the function or dance that people are almost obliged to respect my right to be there. This sort of extrovert behaviour may not be suited to every occasion or applicable for all disfigured people. But the principle is sound: if you display your essential worth and character very positively through your actions, you don't have to depend on your face, your speech or your reputation.

In many ways disfigurement calls for effective acting: your ability to convey more than your looks to your audience is what will influence your reception among them. 'Acting' is sometimes understood to be a superficial way of behaving – people say someone is just acting when they mean he is just putting on some artificial personality. Of course this is not what disfigured people should aim to do – far from it. The acting that is required from you enables your true self to upstage your face. You have to become confident to be seen in public and capable of playing to the gallery – of throwing your personality outwards, literally. This is equally applicable to the physically disabled; anybody whose appearance is discredited has to rely on other forms of communicating their value.

Crowds and public places will pose problems for most disfigured people, but, provided that you do not expect to escape notice and that you are willing to learn and experiment with different tactics, you can gradually regain your poise and come to terms with the inevitable attention you will attract.

CHAPTER 13

With Family and Old Friends

Those who knew you before your facial injury will be in a special relationship with you, as you embark on the process of changing faces. Family and old friends are particularly important in the early, hospital-based part of your recovery, because of the unconditional nature of your relationship with them. By visiting you regularly, they can help you through those painful days and weeks, and, like you, they will be struggling to accept your new appearance and outlook.

They remember you as you were before. They may be horrified at the change. One of my family remembers: 'I had to keep reminding myself that it was *you*. Is it really James? His face has completely changed. I felt miserable with your misery . . . I couldn't tell when you were smiling, so you just looked miserable all the time . . . It must be so much easier for people who had not met you before your accident, because that big adjustment that family, close friends and relatives must go through would not apply.' The extraordinary thing is that the disfigured person is likely to assume just the reverse: you tend to think that while there may be an initial shock, old friends will soon realize that you are still the same behind the scars. But you will probably have to work harder to convince them of this than you would someone completely new who has no adjustment to make. 'Convince' may be a strong word, but old friends are likely to need some help from you, because they have a complex set of feelings to face up to about your new appearance: soul-searching, rejection, total commitment and the other attitudes discussed in Chapter 2. In this chapter I want to concentrate first on two interrelated emotions that people who knew you before may experience: namely nostalgia and reparation. How can you respond to these?

Nostalgia

People who knew you before your facial disfigurement may find themselves thinking about you in rather nostalgic terms. They will be remembering the past and how you used to look, and there will be a hint of sadness in the recollection. Something, they sense, has been lost for ever: your looks, your attractiveness that seemed such an important factor in having a good time and living a full and satisfying life. They wonder if their relationship with you has also seen its best days, and whether it will ever again reach the same heights. It is quite common for this feeling to be experienced by those very close to you – even your wife or husband – because it is really a mourning reaction to your loss.

A classic example of nostalgia is the feelings of an adolescent girl's family after she suffers severe facial injuries: the temptation is for them to think that all the traditional hopes of a happy marriage, etc., have been lost along with her good looks. They may find it very difficult to give her the push and encouragement she needs, being obsessed instead with memories of their earlier hopes for her. Their nostalgia may have undesirable effects on her, because their doubts about her future will allow her to wallow in the past.

Nostalgia essentially hides the fear of old friends that your future is bound to be depressing and painful. It is more comforting for them to remember the good times of yesterday than to face up to the reality of today or the challenge of tomorrow. As the disfigured person, your own determination (or lack of it) to face the future will have a great bearing on how long this nostalgic phase persists. If your approach is forward-looking and you refuse to dwell on past memories, it will rub off on to your friends and family.

Because changing faces is an action-reaction-interaction process, your attitude to yourself will be very much influenced by the quality and quantity of the support given by your close friends and family. In the same reciprocal way, their resolve to look ahead and aid you in your recovery will be to some considerable extent dependent on the determination and perspective you show.

Nostalgia is an inevitable reaction. You too will look back, perhaps, by studying photos of yourself. It is quite difficult to relate to these old photos – somehow they seem to be pictures of someone else – and they have little relevance for the future ahead. I might have been, as one friend described me, 'bronzed, blond, irritatingly good-looking and always pursued by the most attractive girl at the party', but, as he tellingly observed, I was also 'somewhat arrogant'.

Facial disfigurement shatters the idea that your less pleasant personal characteristics can be concealed by good looks. Dealing with nostalgia involves realizing the pretence of your earlier appearance and a readiness to reveal your real personality. Old friends may understandably feel ill at ease if you do start to display parts of your character that you had previously hidden. Your relationship with them was based on something lost, and you may find that they don't want to renew it once they see the new you.

The best plan is to be completely open about what has happened to you behind the scars: your mental approach to the world must change; whereas previously you may have been reluctant to talk about your feelings, now you must be quite prepared to discuss the day-to-day experiences, good and bad, of being disfigured. Your openness and enthusiasm about the challenge of being facially different will help your old friends to understand the new 'you' and see that you are reconciled to a new and positive future.

Reparation

This is a very common feeling among those who knew you before. It is the desire that many people will have to somehow repair your damaged face and restore it to its original shape by making some sacrifice for the guilt they feel. Many a family is struck down by guilt after a fire – even when, as is frequently the case, absolutely no blame can be attached to anyone. Sometimes their guilt gets redirected to someone else who is rightly or wrongly blamed, but too often the family (or one member of it) feel that they have to spend the rest of their lives 'making up for their mistake'. Once they realize that your facial disfigurement is physically irreparable, they may become extremely negative towards you, or, more usually, they may start to give you special treatment to try to compensate you for your loss.

When a child suffers major facial injury, parental guilt may reach such proportions that one or both parents become completely subjugated to serving the child and will give special attention to him as a means of paying off their guilt. The attempt to 'make up for it' is likely to considerably retard the child's process of effectively changing faces, because he will be able to hide behind the feeling that he deserves to be given special treatment. His facial disfigurement will become an excuse for not making anything of his life or for being outside the social and moral requirements of normal society.

If parents do offer 'consolation prizes' and special treatment, there will also be consequences for the rest of the family, who may well end up feeling angry and resentful about the disfigured member's preferential status. Rivalry among brothers and sisters may become intense, and 'normal' children will be confused by the irritation they feel when all the limelight and praise goes to the disfigured child. Yet at the same time they feel guilty about their irritation, because they really want to help in the recovery and show their love.

Family: Your Vital Relationships

Families are put under immense strain by major facial (or other) catastrophes suffered by any of their members. Nostalgia and reparation will come to the surface and may linger too long for anyone's good. It is important that family members and the disfigured person are encouraged to meet and talk about their reactions to the facial disaster. Fortunately, this is now quite high on the agenda of social workers and other carers in hospital burns and facial damage units (see also Chapter 9).

As a disfigured person, you should try to treat your family with the greatest sensitivity. Be aware that their adjustment to your disfigurement may take much longer than you would imagine, and that although their hopes for your facial repair may be quite unrealistic, they will hold on to them desperately. You may have to help them realize that in spite of the slow and limited improvement of your face, your old 'self' remains intact and may even have been matured by your experiences.

In addition to sibling rivalry and resentment that results from excessive parental attention, brothers and sisters, sons and daughters, can react by feeling too embarrassed to be seen in your company. They become afraid to bring friends home, because of the impact a disfigured family member might have on their friendships. Such embarrassment usually indicates that you are being taken at face value by your siblings or children. It may be necessary to help them appreciate the significance of 'appearances are deceptive', and you must be prepared to aid your rehabilitation by informing and spreading positive ideas to other people, their schoolfriends, for example.

While facial disfigurement places immense strains on the family and close friends of its victims, it is important not to dismiss the unexpected gains that are experienced by many families who cope with disfiguring injuries to one of their members. Disfigurement is a crisis, and crises tend to bring people together. The dropping of old family disputes and feuds in the interests of rallying round to help is quite often remarked upon by those who survive major traumas, and usually the strengthened family bonds last well after the immediate recovery stage.

The renewed relationships within your family will be lifted on to a new plane if you can bring yourself to talk about your problems and seek their advice. In this way, relatives can become fully involved in your recovery; and their involvement is needed as much, if not more, after you leave hospital as it is in the early stages of recovery.

Whereas in the hospital setting the onus for opening up new hope may lie with your family, once you are in the public eye it is your initiative that will keep strong family bonds going. It's all too frequent and tragic to see a family rally round in the early days and then fade away once the disfigured person is out in the world again.

Changing faces is likely to involve deepening relationships within your family, but this closeness should not become excessively protective. Sooner or later – and preferably sooner – the disfigured person has to venture out into the world freed from, but buoyed up by, family commitment. Unfortunately, there are examples of disfigured people, especially children, who have been so sheltered from the public gaze by apparently well-intentioned parents or family that they never make the transition to wearing their new face with confidence. This is something that can be achieved only by wearing it in public.

Thankfully, the most common experience is for the trauma of disfigurement to bring out the best in family and victim alike. The crisis triggers off unexpected and unexploited reserves of strength and courage, enthusiasm and laughter. In this atmosphere, changing faces becomes a challenge, not a trial.

CHAPTER 14

Making New Friends

Whatever your age or circumstances, your major difficulty in re-entering the public world after a disfiguring accident, injury or operation is likely to be how to meet new people and become friends with them. Complex as your relations may be with your family and old friends, you will undoubtedly depend on their support enormously until you feel able and/or confident to go back to work, return to college or school, and pick up your life again. As you do this, you will want to establish new relationships, and you may wonder how your face will influence that achievement.

To start with, you will realize that in your days with a normal face, making friends was almost second nature; very little effort was required. If you hit it off with someone, you would become friends, do things together, meet frequently, perhaps confide in each other and generally enjoy each other's company. The starting-point of most friendships is some shared interest or experience. Sometimes one party will 'make the running' – take the initiative to make and maintain contact in order to win over the other. This is just as true whether you have a normal or disfigured face.

Most disfigured people will believe, however, that they start from a disadvantaged position when it comes to making new friends, and that as a result they will have to make *all* the running in trying to build new friendships. You cannot imagine how, with your scars and disfiguring marks, you stand a chance of ever being treated as an equal again, let alone as a friend. And certainly the idea that you might be attractive to the opposite sex will have been almost dismissed from your mind.

You have to face up to this very bleak outlook, but you should not be daunted by it. Within a few days or weeks of disfigurement, you are already making new friends, albeit friends whom you might not have imagined you would meet: nurses, doctors, physiotherapists, ward cleaners and even some of your visitors might be new faces. These new acquaintances should not be dismissed as being just enforced contacts. What you are discovering in going through the agonies of physiotherapy, for example, is that your facial damage does not reduce your interest value. You can have a perfectly worthwhile conversation or interchange of views, and you can still express your feelings of pain or worry and get a response. Your facial injuries may be the reason why you are the subject of a nurse's attention, and in a way a nurse is trained not to notice your injuries. But that is just the point: you are *you*, whatever your face looks like, and that is what the nurse is recognizing: you, face and all.

So, right from the moment of discovering your disfigurement, you should take comfort from the fact that you have not been ostracized and rejected. More importantly, you are at the start of a 'learning process' that will last a long time, possibly for several years. The hospital staff are your first guinea-pigs, and because they will accept you and your new face without reservations, they offer you a unique chance to gain confidence. To some extent the same is true of your family, but the complications of family ties may make confidence-building rather precarious.

The other major consideration that should not escape your notice is that there is only the remotest possibility that any friends you do make will enjoy you for physical appearance alone! Your days of superficial, face-based relationships will certainly be over: friends will now be real friends in that they will have to be prepared to be seen with you and tolerate your scars and misshapen features.

While this is some consolation, it doesn't help you much in actually breaking down the social barriers. You are at a disadvantage, because most people you meet will suffer from one or more ingredients of the SCARED syndrome (see Chapter 10). As I have explained, you cannot allow the SCARED reactions to go unchallenged. They are the first hurdles that everyone you meet has to negotiate. You must be willing and keen to help them to do so.

In many cases, however, your effort may be simply directed to enabling them to overcome their own inhibitions with you, and thus your tactics may not lead to the opportunity for friendships. All you will have done – though it is certainly worth doing – is convey the idea that being disfigured is not the end of the world, and that you are quite sane beneath the scars. A look, a word of reassurance, a moment for them to stare – in these and other ways, you are able to express your humour and humanity.

To go beyond these one-off associations and start to build new friendships will definitely require you to use new skills – communication skills essentially, but you don't have to go off on a course of study in order to gain them. You can learn by trial and error in real life.

The key is to realize that your face begs many questions, but that people you meet will probably have great difficulty formulating the right question. They will be worried about getting the words wrong, about using an inappropriate phrase, about asking too much in case you will find their questions invasive, and much else besides. These worries can prevent them from posing any inquiry at all, and some will just shy away as soon as they feel it is becoming necessary to ask questions about your face. So if you want acquaintances to develop into friends, you have to help them to put their questions. This is a skill that involves perfecting a number of different approaches, then being able to select the appropriate one for the particular person you are with. All the approaches are ways of signalling that you are quite prepared to talk openly about your face if they want to ask.

The least sensitive approach is to launch into a full-scale account of your facial problems before your potential friend has even suggested he would be interested to know more. At the other extreme, you can take the stance of refusing to give anything away at all, believing perhaps that your face is your own private affair. Neither of these methods is likely to win friends. The first assumes that everyone really needs to know about your face, which is definitely not the case and will probably earn you the reputation of being a bore. The second amounts to saying that your face is not socially important – it is and you cannot run from that. Both positions are essentially anti-communication: the first because it swamps your listener and the second because it refuses communication. Changing faces necessitates two-way contact. With possible friends there are three general aids that you can employ to encourage question-asking.

1. In the course of conversation, you can hint that you are quite ready for questions and prepared to answer them. You can do this by casually referring to something medical or to a small part of your recovery. A reference to how you dislike sloppy foods such as semolina after your experience of hospital food can lead on to questions about what happened to you; you can insert a quiet aside about how glad you are that you didn't lose your sight, because you would miss the beautiful scenery; or when talking about phone numbers, you can throw in that you still remember your hospital number.

What you are effectively doing is smoothing out the ground prior to questions being asked and simultaneously offering – not provoking – the chance for your possible ally to take the plunge. Some friends will not feel they need or want to know until really quite long after they meet you and so will turn down your offer. Others will be glad of the opening.

2. You can deliberately see the funny side of awkward situations and in the process shatter any illusions that others may have that your facial looks are a forbidden subject. You will collect quite a repertoire of amusing stories: like the time when a traffic policeman was so baffled by my face that he forgot why he stopped me, or the frequent occasions when people embarrass themselves as they unwittingly comment on how much my son looks like me or they point out the strange reaction of someone else staring at me.

Humour has a great way of breaking the ice and clearing the atmosphere of any trace of embarrassment. It's like a lubricant on conversation and enables you to transmit the message of your willingness to speak openly.

3. A little bit of knowledge goes a long way and sometimes only a small jot of information provided about yourself and your face will put others at their ease. 'I had a car accident' or 'I was burned' might be all that people want to know. Many people are quite content to have gained only a minimal knowledge of your situation and will not need any further details until much later

on in the friendship. Sometimes it amazes me that I have been friends with people for ages and assumed that they have been well-enough informed, when suddenly they pour out a rash of questions like 'We've been meaning to ask for ages . . .'

Facial disfigurement is a very self-absorbing experience and your natural interest in your face and its restoration can blind you to the fact that other people may not share your interest in it. Certainly most friends are likely to comment after knowing you for a while that they don't even notice your face. It doesn't have any bearing on your friendship and little snippets of information are quite enough for them.

That being said, however, there will be people who will help you immensely by allowing you to discharge a lot of your pent-up worries by listening. Having listened, they will never mention the problem again unless you bring it up. Just as it is very important to talk openly to your family when possible, so by talking to friends you can share and be relieved of some of the burdens of disfigurement, as well as receiving whatever reassurance and encouragement you may need.

Your morale will be enormously boosted by encounters with new-found friends that allow you to share your experiences and hear their reactions. Those who knew you before are bound to give a slightly rosy response, one that may be tinged with nostalgia and some guilt even. Someone new with whom you strike up an open friendship allows you to hear for the first time how others see you. Unaffected by your previous reputation, the new friendship starts with no preconceptions, a clean sheet.

New friends will also remind you of a fundamental truth: while you may be very keen to tell all about your rather conspicuous plight and rather nervous about their reaction, they may have a hidden problem of their own that is far more daunting than yours. They may actually need to pour out their anxieties more than you do. Although it can be very inspirational to discover how others have overcome far worse catastrophes than the one that has befallen you, if you do become embroiled with someone who has not really resolved his problem, you may find yourself being dragged into a self-questioning, self-doubting and ultimately self-defeating attitude. You may lose your drive and purposefulness, your resilience may be dented and your risk-taking dulled. Instead of challenging the world, you become daunted by it.

What this warning focuses on is that it matters *how* you talk about your disfigurement and how any new friends respond to it. You will meet those who want to patronize you because they think they ought to do something for someone so obviously unfortunate; you will meet others who may find it hard to live with your frankness and feel unable to offer similar insights into themselves; and you will come across those who almost glorify you on the grounds that you must be such a strong person to have been through your agony. Different people will bring different points of view to bear. All can be friends, and hopefully some will drop their initial reactions and treat you just like any other friend.

Changing faces will necessitate that you relearn how to relate to everybody, including the opposite sex. Your sexual identity will have been shaken, especially if you were young when you became disfigured. You will not form the sort of shallow relationship where facial attraction is the key issue. But worthwhile, lasting relationships depend on the personality as well as the 'packaging'. If you concentrate on coming to terms with your new situation and take up the challenge it offers, you will start to believe in yourself again in a way that makes you a much more interesting person.

The longer you wear your disfigured face the more comfortable you will become with it and the easier it will be to give the right signals and communicate in a straightforward, honest way about your disfigurement. Friendships cemented by that openness will be considerably stronger as a result.

CHAPTER 15

Images of the Disfigured

After the Second World War many men (and some women) who had been facially injured were finding their way back into the public eye. Fighter pilots, naval and tank crews and ordinary civilians all suffered from the rigours of war: fire, explosion, shrapnel and even radiation had damaged many faces. Clubs were established for the veterans who suffered facial fractures or facial burns – the Guinea Pig Club was especially famous as a focal point for men and women recovering from severe burns.

These facially damaged people were a common sight in the years after the war and few ordinary people did not know or know of someone who was recovering. There was a shared appreciation that their facial injuries were indicative of much pain and fortitude: they were brave people who richly deserved the label 'war hero'. A few of them might have appeared on newsreels of the day (shown in cinemas), but the absence of television in no way diminished the high level of public understanding about their plight. More importantly, they were all accorded public respect without question.

Today those who are facially disfigured do not share a common cause. They have been injured or facially operated upon as a result of disparate accidents, disease or misfortune. It is impossible for the general public to identify a single cause for their disfigurement, as they had been able to with the war. After a major accident, a fire at a London Underground station or on a North Sea oil rig, for example, it is some considerable time before the men and women who have suffered serious facial burns re-enter the public domain, and the people they meet will have little memory or understanding of their misfortune.

There is also the added problem that fewer individuals are

likely to know someone who has been facially damaged. However, such is the coverage of television in today's culture that many people will have some awareness of facial disfigurement through the eyes of a camera. There have been some excellent TV documentaries on the subject in recent years: the film about Simon Weston's brave recovery from the fire aboard the *Sir Galahad* in the Falklands' War; the story of David, the Brazilian boy whose face had to be surgically rebuilt after a rare disease had destroyed parts of it; the BBC's *Children in Need* programme in 1988, which contained a lengthy interview with a remarkable girl who had suffered disfiguring birthmarks. And Dennis Potter's drama *The Singing Detective* opened many people's eyes to the problems of psoriasis sufferers. Many of these programmes have mass audiences of ten million or more in Britain and may well have been seen internationally as well. They do much to spread a wider understanding of what disfigurement involves for its victims and their families. The films are sensitive and usually positive, and they do not try to glamorize or overstate the problems. Sometimes a follow-up programme checks on the subject's progress. He is pictured trying to face up to the loss of facial good looks and attractiveness. As individuals, they will win great public sympathy and admiration – rightly so, as apart from anything else they have courageously exposed themselves to media attention.

But do the people who watch the documentaries – and those who don't – instinctively admire and fully accept a disfigured person when they meet one in a public place – a street, a pub, an office? Unfortunately not – and in order to gain that acceptance, you need to appreciate the public's attitude. At times you will even have to justify your existence in the face of public doubts and questions.

Even though people will have an inkling of what Simon Weston, young David, Nikki Lauda, etc., are like via their publicized injuries, I would hazard a guess that all of them are treated as 'odd' in public places. There is still a public uncertainty about their underlying characters. And people who know nothing about *you* will feel equally, if not more, uncertain about your facial impairment.

What lies behind the uncertainty in the way of assumptions

about the facially disfigured as a group? If answers can be found, they will help you to interpret how others are behaving towards you.

Faces are So Important

Of all human physical features, the human face is probably the most significant. The plain fact that you are forced to acknowledge in changing faces is that your misshapen face marks you out from the crowd in a discrediting way.

Some facial features are so highly prized and acclaimed that their owners gain social standing by having them: clear skin and a rosy complexion, bright, well-defined eyes, a shapely nose and a tidy mouth with even white teeth. Other facial features tend to count against you: spots, abnormal growths, a double chin, a large hooked nose. The height and shape of one's figure can also be divided into the socially desirable and undesirable.

People who possess a discrediting feature can become quite obsessed by their irritation with it. Some people take quite drastic actions to remove what they think society devalues: wrinkles, excess fat, etc., can be surgically excised (temporarily). But as has been pointed out previously, the technical brilliance of plastic surgery can never quite renormalize a disfigured face. You will always carry an unusual and remarkable facial appearance.

The human face is the prime canvas upon which each one of us portrays our personality and moods. Through facial expressions – smiling, frowning, grimacing and so on – messages are conveyed to others as regards your emotional reactions and intentions, and as you speak your mouth reinforces the signals. In other words, your face is your major communication device, and in relations with other people you will come to rely on it to say things that can't be transmitted in words.

Disfigurement will distort and disorganize the signalling mechanism: people will unintentionally misinterpret or fail to acknowledge your facial movements. Your smile may be unreachable, and your frown may not have the desired effect.

More important than its value as a signalling box, though, is the face's role in informing others what to expect from the person behind it. As a normal-faced person, you will recall what a buoyant face you presented to the world after a sunny, open-air holiday: you felt healthy and your 'attractiveness quotient' (AQ) – like an intelligence quotient – in the eyes of others probably rose. Your mood and morale were high, and your face was correspondingly that much brighter and more attractive. On the other hand, if you suffered from a bout of flu or cold symptoms, your complexion became pale and pallid, your eyes watery and your AQ will have fallen accordingly. You know then that you are at your least appealing.

Becoming disfigured shatters any pretence you may have had to obtaining a high AQ. You may well have cultivated your appearance very carefully before in order to raise your AQ scores: hairstyling, make-up, a shapely moustache, intelligent-looking spectacles, contact lenses. These are all standard ways of improving your social reception, of making yourself more appealing.

An AQ is literally how much of a magnet your face is. The assumption behind the determined search for higher AQ scores is that by prettying or smartening your face, your social likeability and status rises too. The link between good looks and good character is very strongly imprinted in our culture. So, unfortunately, is the reverse: disfigured looks are frequently associated with less desirable personalities.

The Stigma of Disfigurement

When you face the public, you will be scrutinized and automatic associations will be made in the public mind between your looks and your character. Those connections are rarely flattering, and they will persist unless you challenge them. When a long-standing friend remarked to me that he was glad 'I wasn't as stupid as I looked', what he meant was that there is a commonly held link between rather vacant, expressionless looks and mentally retarded, unintelligent people. In my case he was able to rid himself of that assumption only because he had got to know me. My looks made him think I ought to be low AQ *and* low IQ.

Such a view of the disfigured as stupid, inept or thick is but one of the stigmas attached to disfigurement. To say someone is 'stigmatized' means that he is for some reason disqualified from full social acceptability. In the case of disfigurement, your tarnished face discredits you by automatically casting doubts on your mental ability.

Another frequent association is of disfigured, facially ugly people with some of the more evil characters of fiction, films and children's stories. From a very early age, the imagery of the good with the handsome or pretty, the bad with the scarred or deformed, is imprinted on the public consciousness. The Cinderella pantomime story is a classic case of this, with the Ugly Sisters as the very epitome of nastiness, cruelty, greed, selfishness and exploitation.

If you doubt the widespread acceptance of this sort of stereotyping, you should think of the imagery of horror stories and movies like *Dracula* and *Frankenstein* or the famous villains of literature like Fagin in *Oliver Twist*, described as 'vile and repulsive in appearance'. Children's stories are littered with such symbolism: Peter Pan and his enemy the scary and scarred Captain Hook, the wicked witch in contrast to the spotless Snow White. Nor is adult literature free of stereotyping: *The Hunchback of Notre Dame* and *Dr Jekyll and Mr Hyde* are two striking examples.

It would not matter too much if these over-simple images were effectively overridden by more sensitive images in real life. Unfortunately, they are indirectly strengthened by the pervasive impact of the advertising industry. I am not questioning the purpose of that industry – to promote sales – merely the methods it chooses to employ. The messages attached to any number of advertisements are clever and even insidious, because they play on the glamour and good life that accompanies good looks. Exotic scenes of bikini-clad drinkers of a favourite alcoholic spirit or the jet-setting lifestyle attached to driving the latest sleek motor-car may seem like harmless (if extravagant) ways of persuading people to choose a particular product or brand. Even adverts for humble household cleaning fluids show the perfect loving mother to be blonde, beautiful and blemish-free.

In reality, part of the demoralization felt by the facially impaired stems from the logic behind such adverts. If your face fails to come up to the standards set by the glossy magazines – the cosmetic perfection and the highlighted facial symmetry, for example – your life is doomed, and you have no chance of happiness or success. The stigma implies that the disfigured are bound to be social failures. Although handsome men are similarly stereotyped by adverts, the fact that this logic is particularly devastating for disfigured women is consistently reinforced by the preponderance of advertisements featuring beautiful women.

Another dimension of the stigma is the link between scarred faces and suspiciousness. Scars disturb people's peace of mind, because they suggest links with the criminal classes. The stark (sometimes identikit) pictures of wanted criminals and convicted murderers in newspapers and on television testify to the gaunt and often marked faces of some of the less appealing members of society. Hollywood villains have often been cast in this mould.

Another component of the stigma attached to disfigured people is the presumption that your facial damage indicates that you are in some sense 'unclean'. People who don't have any knowledge of facial injuries wonder whether you may be a carrier of some dreaded infectious disease like leprosy. Will physical contact with you contaminate a normal person or child? While there is a risk in the early, hospital days of facial reconstruction that you may harbour a bacterial infection, it is you who are far more likely to have contracted it from a clean-looking person who has come to visit you with a heavy cold. The unclean association is strengthened by the sanitized and obsessional cleanliness of the advertisers' dream house, food, kitchen, skin, etc. The implication is that if you do possess a blemish, even a little wart, you are less than 100 per cent clean and are therefore some sort of liability and danger to the public.

Dealing with Stigma

The facially disfigured are not, of course, the only group in society to be stigmatized in the public mind: the handicapped, alcoholics, AIDS sufferers, black people, women, even pensioners . . . These and many others suffer from completely unwarranted assumptions about their characters on the basis of some physical or psychological fact about them. Books have been devoted to disentangling these prejudices, and public campaigns are mounted from time to time to try to reduce the public's tendency to impute stigmas. In the case of women and racial prejudice, extensive anti-discriminatory legislation has been enacted in Britain and other countries.

Some of these examples, such as those concerning the advertising industry, may strike you as extreme and far-fetched, but it is as well that as a facially disfigured person you are aware of the possibility that you will be discriminated against by people you meet or pass in public places. The associations of disfigurement with mental deficiency, suspiciousness and/or uncleanliness are well entrenched in today's culture and will not be transformed or eliminated quickly – or, perhaps, ever.

Unfortunately, the stigma does occasionally show itself in acts of unpleasant discrimination towards facial disfigured people. Racial prejudice is much discussed in the media these days, as are sexist attitudes, but the fact that facial prejudice does exist and does lead to unequal treatment of someone because their face bears the marks of an accident or cancer is not perhaps well enough appreciated.

The British media do sometimes make front-page news of such incidents, as they did in late 1988 over the case of a young child with a large strawberry birthmark on his face being ostracized from his playschool because the other children and their parents were apparently upset by his unsightly birthmark. His father complained, 'He's a smashing little boy. The other kiddies weren't bothered. He was just another playmate to them. Now he's been made out to be a leper.' That story hit the headlines, but many small discriminations will go unmentioned: certain jobs, for example, may not be available to the facially injured. Obviously some jobs in the public eye may not be ideally suited for those with damaged faces, but there is no particular reason why this should go completely unchallenged. In my job as a teacher in a girls' secondary school, I certainly try to destroy the myth that disfigurement or disability debars you from doing challenging, intellectual or responsible jobs.

What I have tried to show in this book is that whatever the stigmas surrounding facial disfigurement in the public mind – and they undoubtedly do exist – you can, as an individual, live with and conquer your disfigurement. By watching and talking with others, by acting, reacting and interacting with them, you can re-establish your self-respect. Once you have started to regain your confidence, changing faces can become an interesting and chal-lenging journey for you and others. In your pioneering efforts you will be making the world more tolerable for other facially disfigured people to re-enter and enjoy.

FURTHER READING

Baker, Nancy C., 'The Beauty Trap: How Every Woman Can Save Herself from It', quoted in Marwick, A., *Beauty in History* (Thames & Hudson, London, 1988).

Clinch, Minty (quoting Robert Redford). 'Nice Act. Shame about the Face', *Observer Magazine* (3 April 1988).

Collyer, F. E., *Facial Disfigurement* (Macmillan, London, 1984).

Evans, A. J., 'Cosmetic Surgery of Burns', *British Journal of Hospital Medicine* (June 1981) pp. 547–50.

Goffman, E., *Stigma: Notes on the Management of Spoiled Identity* (Penguin Books, Harmondsworth, 1963).

Hillary, R., *The Last Enemy* (Macmillan, London, 1949), now reissued in paperback (Pan Books, London, 1988). Book 2 is particularly relevant.

Margrave, C., *Cosmetic Surgery* (Penguin Books, Harmondsworth, 1985).

Partridge, James, 'A Patient's Viewpoint of Burns', in P. A. Downie (ed.), *Cash's Textbook of General Medical and Surgical Conditions for Physiotherapists* (second edition, Faber & Faber, London, 1990).

Piff, Christine, *Let's Face It* (Gollancz, London, 1985).

Shakespeare, R., *The Psychology of Handicap* (Methuen, London, 1975).

Sturgeon, D., 'King's Cross Lessons for the Battle against Trauma', *Guardian* (11 November 1988).

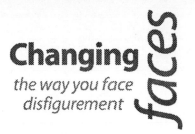

Changing

*the way you face
disfigurement*

Changing Faces is a registered charity, founded in 1992. Its aim is to create a better future for people of all ages who have disfigurements to their face, hands or body from any cause (from birth, accident, cancer, paralysis or skin condition).

Changing Faces

offers one-to-one support, information and advice, especially in social skills training

produces self-help guides for dealing with social situations

promotes holistic health care which recognises the emotional and social aspects of disfigurement

raises public awareness of disfigurement by working with schools, the media and employers

For further information about organisations and groups that support people with different kinds of disfigurement, please visit the *Changing Faces* website where there are many links to relevant organisations.

You can also write to *Changing Faces* if you wish to receive a list of support groups.

For our list of publications and resources or if you would like help or advice about any aspect of disfigurement, please contact us at:

Changing Faces
The Squire Centre
33-37 University Street
London WC1E 6JN
Telephone: +44 (0) 20 7391 9270
Fax: +44 (0) 20 7383 3136
e-mail: info@changingfaces.org.uk
web: www.changingfaces.org.uk

UK Registered Charity No. 1011222

INDEX